WITHDRAWN
WRIGHT STATE UNIVERSITY LIBRARIES

PERSONAL DISORDER
and Family Life

PERSONAL DISORDER
and Family Life

Peter Lomas

Transaction Publishers
New Brunswick (U.S.A.) and London (U.K.)

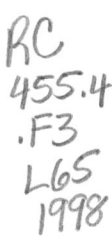

Copyright © 1998 by Transaction Publishers, New Brunswick, New Jersey.

All rights reserved under International and Pan-American Copyright Conventions. No part of this book may be reproduced or transmitted in any form or by any means, electronic or mechanical, including photocopy, recording, or any information storage and retrieval system, without prior permission in writing from the publisher. All inquiries should be addressed to Transaction Publishers, Rutgers—The State University, 35 Berrue Circle, Piscataway, New Jersey 08854-8042.

This book is printed on acid-free paper that meets the American National standard for Permanence of Paper for Printed Library Materials.

Library of Congress Catalog Number: 97–31564
ISBN: 1–56000–341–3
Printed in the United States of America

Library of Congress Cataloging-in-Publication Data

Lomas, Peter.
   Personal disorder and family life / Peter Lomas.
     p. cm.
   Includes bibliographical references and index.
   ISBN 1–56000–341–3 (alk. paper)
     1. Family—Mental health. 2. Family—Psychological aspects.
3. Childbirth—Psychological aspects. 4. Postpartum psychiatric disorders. 5. Psychotherapy—Philosophy. I. Title.
RC455.4.F4L65   1998
616.89—dc21   97–31564
                                                                             CIP

Contents

1. Introduction — 1
2. Family Role and Identity Formation — 11
3. Passivity and Failure of Identity Formation — 29
4. Some Thoughts on Family Relationships in Contemporary Society — 63
5. Family Interaction and the Sick Role — 83
6. Childbirth, the Family, and Breakdown — 91
7. An Approach to a Family Study of Childbirth — 105
8. Observations on the Psychotherapy of Puerperal Breakdown — 125
9. Puerperal Breakdown and Defensive Organisation — 141
10. Dread of Envy as an Etiological Factor in Puerperal Breakdown — 151
11. The Husband-Wife Relationship in Cases of Puerperal Breakdown — 165
12. The Concept of Maternal Love — 177
13. An Interpretation of Modern Obstetric Practice — 189
14. Taboo and Illness — 203
15. Psychoanalysis—Freudian or Existential — 215
16. On Setting up a Psychotherapy Training Scheme — 237
17. The Teaching of Psychotherapy — 247
    Index — 257

1

Introduction

There is no doubt that we are a bewildered society. This is not to say that life is worse for us than in the past, for, in many respects, it is clearly better; but we do appear to suffer from a pervasive ill that is hard to identify. The disease, if such it be, is perhaps nowadays most frequently labelled postmodernism: an abandonment of confident universal beliefs and their replacement by a detached irony. Anthony Giddens, however, persuasively argues[1] that our present state is best described as the consequences of a modernity from which we have not yet escaped, that we are caught up in an age of unprecedented acceleration of change, with ever increasing 'knowledge' of people and their relationships. In such a situation how can we grasp what is going on in the families we study? The families are themselves confused about values and are confronted by a 'generation gap.' And how bewildered by change is the therapist, who not only has to confront what is happening in the family but what is happening in his own discipline. To what extent do Freud's theories still hold? How are his ideas affected by contemporary technology? Freud had no videotape recorder, one-way screen, or computerised methods for organising his material.

It is clear that since that time there has been a development of knowledge gained from dedicated study by some very creative people; Freud's work itself has been closely scrutinised and, in some ways, found wanting. But we are now in danger of losing our way among the legions of theories and techniques that are pressed upon us, and allowing ourselves to become ever more disembodied and afflicted by discontinuity. This does not mean that we should return to Freud anymore than, say, political theory should return to Marx. We have surely learnt that dogma does not get us far. The difficult task seems to be to incorporate the understanding of past workers, even if they come in unappetising styles, and try not to become victims of new dogmas.

In my own training as a psychoanalyst I was fortunate enough to be taught by practitioners who had already moved away from the strictly orthodox view that pervaded most psychoanalytic thinking. They were members of the 'British independent group' or 'object-relations school,' notably Winnicott, Balint, Bowly, Rycroft, and Marion Milner, all of whom had edged away from Freud's instinct theory and opened up a fertile ground for the study of interpersonal relations. Freud's language is still more in evidence in the earlier papers collected here than I now feel comfortable with, but I have only made a few changes to the wording, leaving out, for example, 'a change from object-cathexis to ego-cathexis' which I could no longer stomach in spite of the fact that, in the context of Freud's thought, the words make absolute sense (as is usually the case). I now believe, more than I then did, that any description of psychotherapy is best written in ordinary language, but I hope that these articles are not too afflicted by jargon, and that the valuable ideas I learnt from Freud still hold good.

When we study society and note the phenomenal acceleration of change in recent times it is easy to forget the unchangingness of human nature. Social change has a bearing on the conflicts which the therapist observes in her consulting room, but it does not significantly alter the nature of the child who enters this fragmented world. The discontents of civilisation, the social coercion and the child's revolt against it may take on new forms but the basic conflicts have stability over the generations. Insofar as Freud was right about the elemental familial conflicts that lead to repression or neurosis, he is still right. This line of thought is given support by Galen Strawson, who writes:

> There's a great deal of substance to the idea of a common humanity—of profound emotional and cognitive similarities that transcend differences in cultural experience. It's also true that human beings are very varied, psychologically, but the deepest psychological differences are those that can be found in a given culture.[2]

The universality of human nature does not, however, transcend individuality. Indeed, one of the failings of early psychoanalysis—and, unfortunately, a failing that can still show itself today—was to pay too little attention to the uniqueness of people and the situation in which they live. Most therapists are acutely aware of this uniqueness, but such is the lure of an easy generalisation that students are often taught, and quick to learn and apply, blanket interpretations rather than to search for an intuitive feel of what a patient is really like or what kind of influence has moulded him. In some of what follows here I have attempted to stress this uniqueness. However, given the perennial tension between the universal and the particular, I'd like to address the question: 'How different are the families today from those I wrote about thirty years ago?'

Family constitution is not formed by DNA, yet insofar as families are unities in which child-rearing takes place, they do have something recognisably in common. The society of the eighties and nineties appears, at first sight, to be at the opposite extreme of that of the sixties. Gone are the dreams, the rash ventures into new ways of organising or disorganising life experience, the students who took to the streets rather than studying and planning a career and a mortgage, the drop-outs who disengaged themselves on principle rather than through the exigencies of poverty, and the anti-psychiatrists and gurus. Now we believe in order, control, discipline, adaptation, acceptance and even, in some cases, a return of the 'good behaviour' of the Victorians. If society were a person, and if we held any brief for psychiatric diagnosis, we could say that the 1960s were the age of hysteria and the present age is one of obsessionality.

Yet what similarities are disguised by these impressive differences? The pervasive cynicism about those in power remains, with the difference that there is little belief that anything can be done about it. The phenomenon of the 'absent father,' who appears in so many psychoanalytic case-histories as a force (or lack of force) with immense pathogenic influence on the child, is still a problem. Whereas before he lived at home but put his energy into his work, claiming immunity from such maternal matters as changing nappies, now, although more orientated to child-rearing, he has quite likely departed for another household. And so on. I do not wish to deny the changes or their effects, nor the importance of studying these changes (I have, for example, included here a chapter written on the effect of contemporary hospital regimes on the psychology of the mother and hence on the family as a whole), but I still wish to suggest that those who consult psychotherapists today are beset with the problems that would be easily recognisable by a therapist thirty years ago and would not be incomprehensible in Freud's time.

The more significant question, perhaps, is the degree to which the therapist has changed under the influence of increased experience within her profession and the effect of trends in society. Leaving aside specific issues, however important, (as, for example, attitudes to homosexuality) I would say that the contemporary therapist is less secure in making claims that she knows, better than the patient, how to live. In making this statement I realise I am in danger of putting a point of view which is parochial for I have no access to what goes on in consulting rooms across the country. But I sense, in therapeutic writings at least, a dent in the assurance with which practitioners lord it over their patients in a way that was not uncommon thirty years ago. To set against this trend, however, there is the unhappy prospect that registration of psychotherapists will bring the kind of certainty and assurance that so often accompanies hierarchical institutions whose aim is to achieve the status of expertise for their training and methodology: charismatic power may become displaced by bureaucratic power.

One of the limitations in our understanding of the plight of the contemporary family is the poverty of current sociological research. In the realm of personal experience, sociology, like psychology, has failed us, largely because it tackles questions of immense complexity with undue confidence and relies on quantifications that are too crude. In addition, as Horowitz argues, sociology has forsaken the ethical standards of past major thinkers and, in the United States at least, has been ambushed by those with a vested interest in its conclusions.[3]

Childbirth is the pivotal event for the family, and breakdown after childbirth is a disaster. Yet, when I first sought out the psychoanalytic literature on postpartum breakdown I was dismayed by its paucity. The reason for this neglect, I think, was Freud's patriarchal attitude, lack of interest in the mother's experience, and equation of childbirth with castration. Helene Deutsch wrote well on mothers but was too much a Freudian to escape his perspective and portrayed mother-love as a masochistic phenomenon. Melanie Klein brought the mother well and truly into the picture but only as an 'object' which was the target of infantile projections. It was Winnicott, more than anyone else in the analytic field, who focused our attention onto the experience of the mother and the minutiae of the mother-infant relationships, and who engendered an impressive literature on the subject. Yet, even though postpartum breakdown has received more attention in recent years and been the subject of systematic research[4] it still has not been taken as seriously as is merited by such a devastating event for the family.

The chapters on postpartum breakdown included here were written when I was working at the Cassel Hospital, an avant-garde therapeutic community based on the principles of psychoanalysis, where I had a unique opportunity to study this phenomenon firsthand. The Cassel had its faults. Every incident was analyzed to death. Even the cook was confronted with interpretations about her meals. Tranquilisers were regarded as a short-cut to hell and the taking of an aspirin was a rare and troubling event. But under the dynamic leadership of Tom Main it was an exciting and stimulating place to work in. One of the many innovative policies was to admit mothers suffering from postpartum breakdown together with their babies and sometimes the whole family. Most of the responsibility for this work happened to come my way, and the chapters on postpartum breakdown included here are the consequence of this.

In the last few decades we have been saturated by books, learned papers, and newspaper articles on the problems of the family. There is little agreement about the nature and possible cure for the problem but few are in doubt that the family is in a sorry state. Out of this flood of bewildering hypotheses I would like to select one which has clear relevance to the psychotherapist: the claim that the state has invaded the family to its detriment. There is no doubt that the powers of the family in relation to child-rearing have, in many ways, been eroded. The state has taken over the education of the child and the doctor has assumed the function of health advisor. The ordinary capacities of parents to look after their children, provide moral guidance, and steer them into a place in the outer world has, for various reasons, declined, and experts in these capacities have proliferated. This intrusion into the family has been charted by many thinkers, perhaps most arrestingly in Christopher Lasch's cogent and passionate book 'Haven in a Heartless World':

> Today the state controls not merely the individual's body but as much of his spirit as it can preempt; not merely his outer but his inner life as well; not merely the public realm but the darkest corners of private life, formerly inaccessible to political domination. The citizen's entire existence has now been subjected to social direction, increasingly unmediated by the family or other institutions to which the work of socialization was once confined. Society itself has taken over socialization or subjected family socialization to increasingly effective control. Having thereby weakened the capacity for self-direction and self-control, it has undermined one of the principal sources of social cohesion, only to create new ones more constricting than the old, and ultimately more devastating in their impact on personal and political freedom.[5]

It is ironic that the most powerful influences on family behaviour are the theories of the 'helping professions,' those practitioners (psychiatrists, psychoanalysts, counsellors, and social workers) who are themselves subjected to so much scorn. Yet they have taken on the mantle of the priest and (with the help of sociological theory) replaced the concept of sin with that of sickness and deviance. The criteria of good living is no longer virtue but health and normality. This phenomenon puts psychotherapists in a difficult position: insofar as they claim expertise on the way that individuals and families should behave they are in danger of arrogance and of abusing their powers; insofar as they stress the limitations of their views on how to live they can be accused of failing to give guidance to the family. This dilemma dogs all forms of therapy. When the practitioner moves out of the narrow confines of the consulting room and confronts a family and the social forces that affect a family the risk of making decisions on the basis of an inadequate theory and technique remains high; yet at first sight it may seem that the therapist who moves away from a one-to-one relationship and confronts a family is entering a more ordinary world and will be able to act with more freedom. And, to some extent, this is so. A therapist may visit the family in their home surroundings; people move about and sometimes leave the room, and the therapist is not restricted, as is the psychoanalyst by adopting a self-effacing stance in order that transference will develop. Yet, in spite of this potential freedom, family therapy is even more dominated by technique than individual therapy. To some extent this is to be expected. The family therapist is facing a system rather than a person. She cannot develop the kind of intimate personal relationships which transcend technique (and are all too easily distorted by technique). Indeed, it would be unwise to make a close relationship with one family member in particular. And the mechanical techniques, such as videotape recordings and one-way screens can, to some extent, be justified by the fact that so much is going on in a family session that one pair of ears and eyes is not enough—but it is hard to believe that these measures do not erode spontaneity.

The systemic approach, the history of which, from Bateson onwards, has been admirably documented by Hoffman[6] has, however, proved remarkably creative. What has emerged as a dominant theme, and which appears to practitioners to be of most use, is the development of concepts which help to understand family stasis and to design ways of jolting the family into change. Hoffman likens the situation to that of fishing. 'It is as if a fish, thinking itself quite safe with this booby of a fisherman, suddenly finds itself with a hook in its mouth.'[7] Complicated and desperate manoeuvres occur, but 'the major fact is that the therapist, perhaps for the first time with this family, feels that he has a fighting chance to catch this elusive fish, which is not any particular family member but the relentless pattern that enslaves us all.'

The method—the analysis and confrontation of the defences—is not unlike that of Freud, in spite of the fact that the 'systems approach' is often contrasted with the 'psychodynamic' model. The similarity gives one the thought that, however justified in looking at the problem in this kind of way, and however fruitful it can be, family therapists have become so dependent on their techniques that, like orthodox psychoanalysts, they neglect the innumerable factors, other than a particular theory, that play a part in healing. Ferenczi,[8] who was the leading pioneer in this realm, has not yet been taken with sufficient seriousness. In understanding the factors that help others to live better, either as individuals or families, we have, I believe, a very long way to go.

In both individual and family work a major problem is how to extricate oneself from the powerful influence of Freud, Bateson, and other original thinkers without losing their insights, and incorporate into one's work the values by which we live in everyday life and which can bring a breath of fresh air to musty consulting rooms. Practitioners in both family and individual work, to a varying degree, do bring to their work much that is personal, moral, spontaneous, and intuitive rather than technical; but their theory does not allow for this.[9] Many of the chapters in this collection represent the attempt of one psychoanalyst to free himself from the limitations of a technical way of thinking without impoverishing his work in the process.

Chapter 2 contains the account of the psychoanalysis of a woman considered in the context of her present-day family relationships. When, prior to publication, I read the paper to the British Psychoanalytical Society it was notable how the ideas on family interaction, which I had gleaned from the American studies of Bateson, Wynne, and others, were unfamiliar to a British audience. Psychoanalysis at that time centred almost exclusively on early childhood experience. And, in spite of all that has been written since, individual psychoanalysis has, I believe, still not quite entered the sphere of the patient's everyday life.

Chapter 3 continues the exploration of the family constellation's bearing on a person's sense of identity. The influence of Erik Erikson was then important to me—and continues to be—in understanding the effect of the pressures of family and society on our sense of self. It is surprising that Erikson, whose name was once on everyone's lips, has fallen so much into the background.

Chapter 4 extends the discussion to include the place of the family in society, while still incorporating psychoanalytic and family therapy concepts. In revising this paper, written thirty years ago, it is all too obvious that the problems which beset families in our culture have, as I suggested above, changed little. We seem, in spite of our research, to be in little better shape in knowing how to bring up children and steer them through the pitfalls of rivalry and disillusionment which Freud outlined a century ago. We need, I believe, to take another look at Dewey, Montessori, Froebel, and other seminal thinkers on child rearing.

Increasingly, both in individual and family work, I have come to realise the centrality of power relations. Chapter 5, 'Family Interaction and the Sick Role,' incorporates ideas derived from Balint, Main, and Szasz, and attempts to spell out the ambiguities of power and weakness constitutive of the person who claims, or is deemed, to be sick. It is a theme to which I return in chapter 14, 'Taboo and Illness.'

Chapters 6–13 all focus on childbirth and its psychological exigencies. In 'The Concept of Maternal Love' I criticise Freud's very negative view of childbirth, a view which, though generally accepted by psychoanalysts at the time, is a strikingly bizarre one. It was surely one of Freud's greatest errors of judgement to denigrate the act (a'castration') which results in a new human being. One of the most vivid memories I retain from the time when I was a general practitioner is the feeling of transcendence that so often pervaded everyone present on the occasion of a successful birth at home. Although these chapters undoubtedly were provoked by working at the Cassel Hospital with mothers who had broken down, my interest in the subject could hardly be unconnected with my being a parent of young children at the time that I was writing. Indeed, the research which I undertook with my wife, Diana (some of which is included in chapter 7), owe much to her maternal intuition.

Chapter 15 is an attempt to formulate the relationship between Freud and Existential psychoanalysis. There is far more agreement between the Existentialists and the British 'Independent' School of thought than the latter seem able to recognise. I suspect that the perennial loyalty to Freud has stood in the way of this recognition, as, unhappily, it has done in so many areas of thought.

The final two chapters are about the teaching of psychotherapy and are based, in part, on the experience of some of us who have attempted to provide a training for students which departs radically from the currently accepted format. The organisation, namely, the Cambridge Society for Psychotherapy, provides a setting in which students, both individually and collectively, take responsibility for their own training, thus giving them the possibility of finding whatever style of learning, thinking, and practice is most suitable to their personal make-up. At the time I wrote these papers I expressed a fear that our greatest obstacle would be the pressure to conform to the required standards of the recently formed Register of Psychotherapists. Unhappily these fears were all too realistic and we have found it difficult to maintain integrity and creativity in the face of external pressure. I was much encouraged by reading Otto Kernberg's ironic, wise and engaging paper, published recently, 'Thirty methods to destroy the creativity of psychoanalytic candidates.'[10] I rather doubt, however, whether the article will be taken as seriously as it is meant to be.

When I look for a central theme which persists throughout the chapters in this book it seems to be a concern with those factors which inhibit the development of a sense of personal responsibility, whether it be the patient in the consulting room, the child in the family, the mother in the maternity hospital or the student in training. The factors are many and include the individual's tendency to retreat into passivity, the greed and lust for power which divides the world into winners and losers, and the widespread belief that there are people around who possess an expertise in the art of living which justifies their attempt to prescribe for others.

Since writing several of these chapters I have stopped calling myself a psychoanalyst. This does not mean that I wish to renounce my enormous indebtedness to Freud or disown anything that is written here, but that I now feel uncomfortable with Freud's system of thought, technique of therapy, specialised language, and an air of certainty. I find that I can more easily feel at home with those who, like Tolstoy, believe that theories intended to explain our way of living fall abysmally short of doing so for they cannot encompass the infinite variety and detail which human beings encounter.

References

1. Giddens, A. (1990), *The Consequences of Modernity*, Polity Press, Cambridge.
2. Strawson, G. (1996), 'The Sense of the Self,' *New York Review of Books*, 18 April.
3. Horowitz, I.L. (1993), *The Decomposition of Sociology*, Oxford University Press, Oxford.
4. Raphael-Leff, J. (1991), *Psychological Processes of Childbearing*, Chapman & Hall, London.
5. Lasch, C. (1995), *Haven in a Heartless World*, Norton, New York and London, p. 189.
6. Hoffman, L. (1981), *Foundations of Family Therapy: A Conceptual for Systems Change*, Basic Books, New York.
7. Ibid. p. 328
8. Ferenczi, S. (1988), *The Clinical Diary of Sander Ferenczi*, edited by J. Dupont, translated by M. Balint and N. Jackson, Harvard University Press, Cambridge, MA.
9. Lomas, P. (1994), *Cultivating Intuition*, Jason Aronson, Northvale, NJ and Penguin, London.
10. Kernberg, O. (1996), 'Thirty Methods to Destroy the Creativity of Psychoanalytic Candidates,' *Int. J. Psychoanal.* 77, 1031.

2

Family Role and Identity Formation

In this chapter a patient will be described whose illness can be best understood as a failed attempt to establish an identity of her own as opposed to one thrust upon her by her family's need.

Miss F. came to analysis at the age of thirty, having been psychiatrically ill for six years. Her main presenting symptoms were phobic, and included fears of travelling and of being poisoned. Both fears were very incapacitating and resulted in an inability to work. She lived with her mother and father, never went out except occasionally to the local library, and could not eat or drink anything that her mother had not first tasted. She attended for treatment in a taxi, accompanied by her mother.

Her greatest fear was of blindness, and she was also afraid of insanity and was unsure of the correctness of her perceptions. She had been temporarily certified once on account of an anorexia nervosa which endangered her life, and had spent several months in a mental hospital. She thought that at times she had had visual hallucinations, but remained uncertain about this.

In appearance Miss F. was a tall, gaunt woman with long hair who walked in a disjointed way as though liable to fall to pieces; it was difficult to imagine her as the successful model she had once been. Her anxious and rather haggard face readily broke into a charming smile, and she talked incessantly and irrepressibly in a pleasant upper middle class voice. She was untidily dressed and her clothes were dirty.

Originally published in the *International Journal of Psychoanalysis* (1961), 42, 372.

The Family

Her parents were working-class country people who came to London soon after they were married. The husband had completed his apprenticeship as a butcher, and had the prospect of a good job, but was persuaded by his wife to abandon this and to move to London because her own brothers and sisters were migrating there. They came to live 'below stairs' in a West End house where the wife acted as housekeeper; the husband took employment as a railway porter.

One effect of this move was to instil into the family a feeling of inferiority. The wife identified herself with the social behaviour of the family upstairs and strove to emulate it, while at the same time accepting her inferior position. She altered her speech, sought to efface any trace of her West Country upbringing, laid great emphasis on nice manners, and tried to make herself invisible in the presence of her employers.

The husband on the other hand denied any feeling of inferiority, loudly pronounced himself a 'common working man and proud of it,' and would flaunt his broad accent and his porter's uniform whenever possible, an attitude which caused his wife agonies of embarrassment and shame. In this way an ever-increasing rift developed between husband and wife, and it was into this family configuration that the patient was born. She was an only child.

She describes her father as a childish, irritable, pompous man who drank and strutted about, but was dominated by his quietly subtle and persistent wife who was overtly subservient to him, but in matters of importance took no notice of his views. The father became increasingly less of a force in the household. He allowed himself no social ambitions and saved no money. The mother on the other hand carefully saved her earnings and ended up by buying a new house, thus moving into a position of independence and power.

The Patient's Relationship with her Parents

For session after session Miss F. let forth a tirade of abuse about her father. Her complaints about him centred on his interference with her and domination over her. What she most despised and hated was the hypocrisy and pomp (at which her mother connived) with which he kept up a pretence that he was an important being worthy of great respect. This, she felt, might have been tolerable if he had not been a fake.

The role that she was supposed to play as a loving daughter was a result of the insecurity of the family as a whole. Thus her mother defensively tried to establish a rigid family pattern of mutual loyalty in order to combat the feared dissolution of the family owing to the husband-wife split. The daughter was treated as a symbol of family unity and it became desperately important, particularly to the mother, that she fulfil this role. Added to this she had to be the well-behaved landlady's daughter who knew her place. It was well brought home to the patient by the mother's anxiety that if she stepped out of this role the family would collapse and with it the patient's life, for it was part of the family system that the daughter have little outside life.

What seemed to be most disturbing to the patient was the superficial acceptance as true of a false situation and a denial of emotional reality. The myth of a united family was propagated both inside and outside the home. Miss F. described with rage and contempt the Sunday afternoon walks in the park, herself between her parents, her father with a smile of genial protectiveness and her mother looking meek and good. The patient felt imprisoned within this myth and helpless to destroy it; yet to destroy it seemed absolutely vital to her, and she despaired that everyone outside was taken in by it. In her teens she remembers praying that her father might be arrested for drunkenness or develop d.t.'s. Then she would be able to say: 'Look! I am *not* a bad child; it is my father who is mad.' As a child she had been unable to challenge the family myth directly at all and opposed it only by neurotic symptoms. As she grew up, however, she gradually attacked it at its weakest link, her father, in forceful tirades against his attempts to dominate her.

The basic marital disharmony resulted in each of the parents seeking the patient as a loved object to supplant the marriage partner, with the result that the patient had to fulfil another role and one which conflicted with that of a good and innocent child, symbol of family unity. Her resentment at her father's attempts to dominate and discipline her was surpassed by her resentment at his jealous devotion. He was very jealous of her affection for her cat and could not bear her to stroke it in his presence; in various ways he showed his sexual interest in her. It seemed that he wanted from her the sexual and maternal love he failed to get from his wife.

Miss F. suffered from an extreme fear of men and at thirty was a virgin. This fear derived from oedipal guilt feelings and from her projected aggression due to envy of men (an envy fostered by her parents' official doctrine of Victorian morality in which the woman's role was supposed to be that of a household drudge subservient to the man), but also from the threat to her sense of identity if anyone laid a claim to her. Her anger at her father's interest was really vicious: 'He should have been castrated!' she would scream. In a general sense she had in fact succeeded in doing this, using her illness as a weapon. One of her symptoms was a need to be with her mother, a need with which her mother in turn willingly colluded owing to her own frustrated wish for a love-object. The result of this was that the father was gradually ousted and at the time of treatment lived away from home except at weekends and appeared to have no rights whatever. But this success did not at all assuage the patient's wrath, partly because she had displaced her anger over her mother's domination (which was very real and massive) onto her father.

Her relationship with her mother was a more clearly ambivalent one, but the real basis of the feelings involved was hidden. In all small matters she fought for her rights and by her illness compelled her mother to orientate her life around her, and to work herself to the bone in order to pay for her treatment. But in the major issue of developing independent and adult status the patient gave way to her mother's unconscious possessive demand. She had never, for instance, washed her own clothes. It became clear how much this was out of fear of her mother's need to do the washing herself as a symbol of possession, and, when she began for the first time, during the course of treatment, to do some of her own washing it was only in secrecy when her mother was out.

This parasitically symbiotic relationship was of the kind that typically occurs between a 'schizophrenogenic' mother and her daughter, one of the features of which is that the mother's greedy possessiveness is not overt but is concealed under a cloak of interest in the daughter's well-being. This concealment resulted, in the relationship under study, in some rather strange compromises. When the patient succeeded, for the first time in her life, in being away from home, this was not quite the successful emancipation it might appear to be, for she lived in lodgings in the next street and the mother insisted on carrying round fully cooked meals in a suitcase daily to help fatten up her daughter, who eventually was shamed into giving up this venture. The daughter took refuge in a 'flat' in the attic of her parent's house, and had a lock and key installed, but the key was soon lost and her attempt at privacy was frustrated. Moreover her mother became ill from going up and down stairs, and the daughter eventually gave up her flat also. In these manoeuvres the daughter unconsciously colluded with her mother, partly because she had been seduced by secondary gains and partly out of a need to conform.

Miss F. remembered, however, one occasion in her adult life when the tyranny of her mother's possessiveness broke through the mask of benignity. This occurred when the patient, taking a long time to wash in the bathroom, was asked by her mother to hurry up in order to go out with her. The patient, for once claiming privacy, stubbornly locked the door, whereupon the mother, forgetting her gentility and the people upstairs, screamed and threatened and beat upon the door with such ferocity that the panel cracked. This cowed the daughter, who then opened the door.

The Patient's Behaviour during Analysis

It is not my intention in this chapter to discuss treatment, but it is necessary to refer to the patient's analysis in order to fill out the description of the case.

She came to me after having had four years' treatment with a previous therapist to whom she had applied for help when, during her period of modelling work, she had developed incapacitating anxiety attacks and travel phobia. The treatment had been by no means a success; during it she had developed anorexia nervosa and had had two sojourns in mental hospital. Her therapist's technique had consisted of a mixture of interpretation and authoritarian persuasion, and she had reacted to the latter with a revolt and hatred which finally led her to attempt a lawsuit against him.

For the first six months of analysis a large proportion of the time was spent in her description of the differences of opinion between her previous therapist and herself, and her attempt to persuade me to arbitrate in her favour. Her fear and anger towards him were mainly on account of his attempts to 'indoctrinate' her, or 'mould' her according to his moral beliefs, and finally his commitment of her to a mental hospital against her wishes. I was soon to learn that this terror of indoctrination extended to all spheres of her life and showed itself in her relationship with me. She had come to analysis with mistrust and fear and only as a last desperate resort. She had a series of nightmares in which she was misunderstood, disbelieved, certified, locked up or leucotomized by me or by other psychiatrists, although in her waking life she idealized me and could not understand these thoughts. This fear of me became so great that finally she was unable to visit me even with her mother in the waiting room and the taxi and driver outside—at the ready as it were. The treatment was continued by correspondence, but she had a similarly powerful fear that her letters would be taken by me as suitable evidence to certify her. Eventually I came to treat her at home where, in her familiar surroundings, she felt a certain security against me. Other factors entered into her wish to be treated at home—a grandiose wish to be the Queen-Baby who was waited on by me, and a need to defer (in her mind at any rate) to her mother's need to keep her at home as a helpless (child) invalid.

At no point in the treatment was it possible for me to mould her to my own way of thinking, for she made it quite clear by actions as well as words that she was only interested in an attempt at cure that respected her own right to live as she pleased. She was also very concerned that between us we get at the truth, being quite often much more meticulous than I at exploring every possible channel of misunderstanding before considering an interpretation. Inevitably, of course, her passion for truth failed her where her deepest resistances lay. This occurred particularly in relation to feelings of guilt, and it was a long time before this subject could be discussed with any coherence. Her reluctance to consider guilt feelings lay mainly in the fact that she feared being unable to distinguish between 'real guilt' and 'indoctrination guilt.' (It was clear that she had been subjected to plenty of the latter as a child and she recalled, for instance, how she had been told in her teens that if she was unkind to her mother when she was menstruating she—the mother—might die).

In general, the outstanding feature of her behaviour in analysis was a despairing uncertainty about her perceptions (both physical and moral), a bitter anger if they were challenged, and an urgent need to have them ratified by an impartial person. On one occasion she said: 'If you had told me that yesterday you wore a false beard I should not know whether you were telling the truth or not'; and on many occasions she appealed to me to verify not only her moral and aesthetic perceptions but her physical ones as well. These doubts were clearly linked to her fear of insanity.

In an effort to counter her doubts of her perceptions she had developed a capacity for thought that was unusually effective except in the areas in which it was blocked, and a sensitive perception which was rather formidable. She could also muster an extraordinary persuasiveness, a capacity of which she was aware with a mixture of pride and fear. 'I could always sell anybody anything,' she said, and as a model she had been conspicuously successful in selling her appearance.

Because of this capacity to bewitch it was always a precarious undertaking to attempt to estimate the truth of her statements. Moreover, she projected this capacity and consequently felt that others were trying to confuse and bully her, and it was difficult to assess the degree to which her accusations were based on this projection. However, her verbatim reports of her dealings with other people bore the stamp of spontaneity and truth, and I recognized in the reported reactions of these people my own counter-transference. This particularly occurred when I found myself tending to react to her insinuating forcefulness with the same mixture of benevolent acquiescence and sudden authoritarianism as she had portrayed her previous therapist's response.

Closely linked with her fear for her perceptual ability was that of a failure to establish herself as an individual who existed in her own right and not as a standardized and soulless unit of society.

The Effect of the Family Organisation on the Patient's Sense of Identity

According to Erikson[1] the term identity 'connotes both a persistent sameness within oneself (self-sameness) and a persistent sharing of some kind of essential character with others.' He also writes: 'While the end of adolescence thus is a stage of an overt identity *crisis*, identity formation neither begins nor ends with adolescence: it is a lifelong development largely unconscious to the individual and his society. Its roots go back all the way to the first self-recognition: in the baby's earliest exchanges of smiles there is something of a *self-realization coupled with a mutual recognition.*'

In keeping with Erikson's formulations the term *identity* will here be used to connote a 'self-sameness' based both on self-perception and on a comparison with and recognition by the environment (in this case we shall be mainly concerned with the family).

Miss F.'s ability to form an identity was threatened in several ways, which, although interrelated, will for convenience be dealt with separately.

1. Her ability to perceive herself and to trust in herself as an organism with stability of perception was interfered with by the falsifying of emotional reality that occurred in the family.
2. She was unable to find, in her environment, a person or idea with whom or with which to identify.
3. Because she was being used to propagate a family myth and not as a real person there was a confusion between her self-perception and her perception of herself as seen in the eyes of her family.

To take these in order:

1. A stable and coherent presentation of reality is necessary for a child to acquire belief in his capacity for reality-testing. Reality as presented by Miss F's family was unstable because the parents were divided and confused, and because they confused her in their attempts to preserve themselves. What particularly angered the patient was that her mother would not admit any contradictions but would blandly deny what she had previously said. She would agree with her husband's views when he was present, act in opposition to them when he was absent, yet deny the contradiction. Her attitude to her daughter's sexuality was surprisingly inconsistent. Having brought her up to believe in gentility and chastity she suggested on one occasion that she take a rich lover to help out funds.

It was the patient's belief that her mother's method of maintaining discipline was based on an attempt to confuse her and to make her lose her confidence by instilling a belief that she was not understandable, was uniquely naughty, and heading for insanity. Such an attempt to drive the other person crazy has been the subject of a recent paper by Searles[2] and such methods in varying degree of intensity are not perhaps unusual types of domestic discipline.

2. For a philosophy of life she was presented with the choice of the 'upstairs' gentility of her mother or the common working man downstairs, and she was torn between the two. Both had their disadvantages. Although, like the mother, she admired and envied the riches,

the comforts, and the quiet of upstairs life it remained an unrealistic dream; moreover she had great difficulty in identifying with her mother who represented the Victorian, desexualized, downtrodden woman who served her Master. Her father also subscribed to this view. 'A woman is only beautiful' he would say, 'when she's scrubbing the clothes and covered with sweat.' Moreover she could neither easily identify with nor react to the coarse and pompous virility of her father, who would shout, spit, and exhibit his bodily functions, provoked to defiance by her mother's asceticism.

The unhappy compromises in sexual identity formation may well have had psychosomatic results, for her breast development was completely lacking. Her description of herself as 'flat as a pancake, with a beak of a nose, a face like a horse, and legs hairy as a prize-fighter's chin' was an unkind one, but it must have required a remarkable tenacity for this woman to have become a successful model.

3. Wynne et al.[3] describe a certain type of mechanism, called by them 'pseudo-mutuality,' which they have found to occur in the families of patients who suffer from acute schizophrenic episodes. According to them this mechanism occurs in other families but with less intensity. Pseudo-mutuality consists of a relationship in which the person is not treated as an individual in his own right but as having a certain family role. Families in which this occurs are characterized by 'a predominant absorption in fitting together, at the expense of the differentiation of the identities: there exists intense pseudo-mutuality there develops a 'particular variety of shared family mechanisms by which deviations from the family role structure are excluded from recognition or are delusionally re-interpreted. These shared mechanisms act at a primitive level in preventing the articulation and selection of any meanings that might enable the individual family member to differentiate his personal identity either within or outside of the family role structure.'

Miss F.'s family showed many of the characteristics of pseudo-mutuality, and, although she did not develop an acute schizophrenic episode, her psychopathology, particularly the intense idealization and splitting mechanisms, came near to that of a schizophrenic type, and her incapacity to deal with the world in a realistic way approached psychotic intensity.

One of the features of this type of family is that it remains static and does not allow for change; the child is not allowed to grow up. This was certainly true of Miss F., who was her mother's child at thirty and who complained bitterly that in her teens her mother dressed her in clothes too young for her, made her play with younger children, and discouraged sexual development. One got the impression, too, that she had never been allowed to be a real baby. She described herself as a precocious child, who nevertheless was later surpassed by her school friends. It seems from this that her role in the family pattern was that of a child of the latency period and that she was allowed neither to be a baby at the right time nor to grow up.

This rigid family role would seem to be likely to lead to the development of a 'pseudo-self' or 'false-self' as conceptualized by Winnicott.[4] The patient's concern for her true self is depicted in one of her dreams. She dreamed that visitors came to the family. She held a baby in her arms. It was considered important by her mother in order to impress the visitor that the baby sit at table. Miss F. knew the baby was too young to do this but was carried away by her mother's earnestness and attempted it. The baby fell down and broke its skull. Her mother told her to put it outside, which she did, but felt very guilty and concerned about the baby. The baby seems to represent herself who had been prematurely forced to grow up, and adopt a 'false self,' yet preoccupied with the 'true self' which had been left behind. Winnicott believes that the false self develops as a result of faulty early handling by the mother and consists in an attempt on the part of the baby to take over the mothering function. It would seem, however, that the total family configuration also plays a part throughout the child's upbringing in helping to establish a real individuality.

The Patient's Symptoms

By various splitting mechanisms the patient had become able to accept a position of subjection in which her individuality was disregarded and she remained helplessly tied to her mother, while in certain spheres desperately attacking any trace of possible subjection, and asserting her individuality strenuously. During the war, for instance, she refused to do any war work, feeling it to be an infringement of her rights, and she would argue for hours against imaginary disciplinarians who would force her to love, to work, to have children, or to be 'normal' in any way. It seemed likely that this was the origin of her fears of death, insanity, blindness, brain-washing, confinement, hypnosis, rape, castration, poisoning, and so forth—all of which represented in some way an annihilation of her identity or the forcing on to her of an alien identity. What she avoided by these splitting mechanisms was a recognition of the intense hate she felt, particularly towards her mother, on account of the suppression of her individuality.

Miss F. was breast-fed and had a mental picture of herself as a baby growing fatter and fatter while her mother became correspondingly worn and thin and ill. This well depicts one aspect of her relationship with her mother, for she ruthlessly exploited her mother's capacity for masochistic care. Her paranoid fears of control by various means were the result of a vicious circle of mutual parasitism, for the more she feared control the more greedy and controlling she became in self-defence. It is difficult to be certain of the starting point of this vicious circle. The family configuration described would have been likely to suppress the patient's expression of individuality from the start of her life, but presumably this would not have been of such importance to her during early infancy provided basic biological needs were satisfied. That they were satisfied is suggested by the fact that she was breast-fed 'much longer than is usual' and that she was a 'bonny, bouncing baby.' Moreover she was also said to be a 'beautiful baby, with bright blue eyes and long eyelashes' who was doted on by all her relatives and smiled upon by strangers. It may be that her very early experiences were relatively good and gave her the belief in life which she still has and helped to insure her against schizophrenia.

The patient's fear of insanity is of central importance, for it would seem to be the most direct manifestation of her fears. It is perhaps true to say that fear of insanity is the conscious expression of an unconscious fear of loss of identity. Sanity, like identity, has two aspects: the coherence of inner feelings and perceptions of the individual and the recognition of this coherence by society. Complications arise to the extent that society is not coherent, and in the case described, society, as represented by the family, was not. The patient was, then, left with the dilemma of losing belief in her real self and her own perceptions and accepting the pseudo-identity thrust upon her by the family (which represented insanity through perceptual failure) or of accepting her own perceptions as real and risking being thought insane by the family. It was this dilemma that she sought to resolve in her analysis.

This non-logical and unrealistic splitting of reality, impossible to resolve owing to blurring and denial, inevitably resulted in a corresponding splitting and confusion in the patient's own psyche, a process which was elaborated by her own defence mechanisms of denial and idealization.

Thus there were three ways in which she felt her sanity threatened:

1. by adoption of a pseudo-sanity;
2. by being thought insane by society;
3. by confusion, resulting in a complete breakdown of logical thought and a regression to primary process thinking—insanity proper.

Like Shaw, who was 'born mad or a little too sane,' and who remained 'a sojourner on this planet rather than a native of it,' she found affinity only with the 'mighty dead.'[5] This is rather surprising in that, unlike Shaw, she showed no sign of creative talent—at least not until her mid-twenties. It is significant that she identified herself with those great artists who lost their perceptive functions of sight or hearing.

The Patient's Creative Urge

The only evidence Miss F. could give me of a creative urge in childhood was the memory of proudly distributing her faeces around her father's tomato plants in the greenhouse in the hope of making them flourish. She did, however, daydream a great deal and thought that her dreams would become reality, not by realistic effort but by some kind of magic; a thought which was frightening to her. Her night dreams were very vivid and sometimes resembled artistic creations; she took an almost aesthetic pleasure in relating them, although most of them were terrifying.

When she was twenty she trained as a model. She was a very bad pupil, being quite unable to learn from the teacher, but after slowly and laboriously teaching herself she eventually became quite successful. She did not regard this work as creative, but it seemed to me to be an attempt to create a new self, totally unrelated to that which consisted of an adaptation to family role pattern—a glamorous, sophisticated, emancipated, and sexual woman. But this role was too alien to that demanded by her upbringing for her to be able to bridge the gap, and caused her too much guilt, and it was while she was working as a model that she fell ill.

Her next attempt at creativity was more successful. She trained in the making of artificial flowers, and just as during her course of training as a model she could not learn from the teacher but had laboriously to teach herself. The end result was, as in the case of her modelling, very successful insofar as the product was concerned. Her flowers were admired by everybody and even held in awe by the teacher. They looked like real flowers. But this occupation too proved disastrous. She began to believe that her flowers rivalled those of God; she had to cease this work, and fell into a dangerous state of anorexia nervosa. This was the end of her creative efforts—efforts which seemed to derive from a need to attempt to establish a sense of identity which could not be established as a child.

One feature of her creative attempt was a need to do it in her own time. This applied not only to the flower work but to everything in her life, and of course constituted a problem in her analysis. It was in part a consequence of her mother's anxious and hasty method of upbringing. The patient herself, although born in London, never accepted the bustle of City life and yearned nostalgically for the slower tempo of the life of her grandparents in the West Country. (It was as though the clan experimental migration had failed and Miss F. constituted its failure.)

Marion Milner[6] compares the artist's use of his medium—the 'intervening substance through which impressions are conveyed to the senses'—with the use a child made, during analysis, both of herself and the playroom equipment. If such a medium is pliable the child can project his fantasies onto it and can allow a temporary merging of the boundaries between self and not-self, a process that is necessary for reality testing and personality growth. This concept of medium can also be usefully applied, with quantative changes, to the social milieu or total area of communication in a family system which gives each member his life-space, and such a medium can be seen to be necessary not only to the young child but the adult. Perception is itself a creative process and depends not only on the ability to receive the immediate stimulus from the environment but to stand apart from the stimulus and from a rigid mental set from which to view it and to form an impression made fresh and rich by the use of imagination. In a flexible family system based on real communication and the accurate perception of reality, the individuals are sufficiently well-defined and secure to be capable of imaginative perception, to present themselves coherently to others for inspection, and to allow others enough room for them to be able to make this inspection with the full use of their mental powers. The individuals are also capable of fusing together into a viable and changing system of object-relationships—the family—which is itself a creative achievement.

By contrast, in the family structure under study no such medium by means of which the patient could communicate herself in a meaningful way to her parents was permitted, precisely because of the parents' belief that such communication would destroy the family myth. Creative union was replaced by confusion—the superimposition of contraries without attempt to integrate into a new pattern. The life-space of each individual was restricted, autonomy was at a minimum, and communication occurred not between real people but between falsely represented personalities living parasitically on each other by the use of identificatory mechanisms. Miss F.'s creative efforts caused her so much anxiety and guilt because they represented an attempt to communicate her real self, an undertaking which if it had been successful in her childhood could have destroyed the family role identity imposed on her and with it the whole family system; they contained all her destructive and constructive wishes to reorganize the world according to her own ideas. In this way her dream would become reality and God (her father) would be destroyed. (As I have indicated, she had been fairly successful in the destructive aspect of this wish towards her father.) Thus her fears were, to an extent justified; not only was her family unstable and an effort towards individuality and spontaneity on her part would have been liable to wreck it, but she had the capacity to do this in a not very obvious way, for she was a very intelligent girl, probably with much greater perceptive ability than her parents; and she had a peculiar witch-like capacity of persuading and influencing which was difficult to withstand. This can be thought of as an ability to impose her dreams, wishes, and opinions onto other persons so that they accept her view of reality and give up their own. It was a constant fear of the patient that she would drive me insane, and although my countertransference anxieties were not quite of this severity I soon discovered that she was more able to affect my judgement than were my other patients.

There was another way in which the pseudo-mutuality of this family hindered her creative efforts. The way to real development taking place within object relationships being barred and activity being restricted to family role behaviour, the only apparent means of development would be to interchange roles. It was clear that the father and daughter attempted to do this: the patient felt his rivalry to be that of another child and resented her mother pandering to his childish temper tantrums; and she certainly ended up victor in this struggle. But she could never attempt to usurp the father in his role as man of the house, or that of her mother as the woman. Hence her wishes to mature in a feminine way meant to her the usurping of her mother's position. (The apparent necessity to steal another's role in order to make an emotional advance within such a family structure may be a contributing factor in the wish of the child to kill its parent described in the classical Oedipus complex.) Thus it made her feel guilty to create flowers not only because this symbolized the destruction and reconstruction of the rigid family system but because it also represented her wish to become a woman, which involved the usurping of her mother's role. The making of flowers better than real flowers also brought her into direct rivalry with her father in quite a simple way. He was a great gardener and was always 'dragging out' the family to admire his wonderful flowers. Creative work was undertaken by the patient not only for its essentially positive elements but in a defensive attempt to free herself from the narcissism of her parents and bring them to submissive adulation of the glory and importance of her own work. She elevated her work to that of a God.

Conclusion

An attempt has been made to describe this patient's illness in terms of the failure of a family organization. This is not to say that the early physical handling of the patient, or the vicissitudes of her instinctual drives, were not regarded as important or did not come into the analysis, but rather that when they were important they could usually be seen to be related to the family pattern. For instance, that repression of her aggression resulted in paranoid fears could be seen from a study of her many dreams; often she dreamed of domesticated animals with whom she was identified and who became wild and frightening and who attacked her. But the domesticated animal represented the self as it was designated by the family role structure, a self which felt imprisoned and tormented with rage at its impotence. And the paranoid fears represented not only projected aggression turned against the self but an estimation of the actual anger that would have been unleashed by her frightened parents had she revealed her thoughts.

The essence of this patient's illness lay in her difficulty in establishing a sense of individuality. Some of her symptoms—perceptual failure, pathological dependence, inhibition of aggression and sexuality, and self-destructive tendencies—represented the attempt on the part of the superego (in particular as far as it was derived from an internalization of the family system) to suppress individuality; other symptoms—paranoid anxieties concerning death, blindness, castration, suffocation, and poisoning—expressed her fear of the annihilation of her individuality; her chronic ill health and mental and physical delicacy embodied an attempt to find a spurious identity based on her status as an invalid requiring special consideration[7]; her creative urge resulted from a positive wish to establish an individuality if only in a localized sphere, and symbolically. The word individuality is here used to mean a sense of uniqueness, a personal identity that is not derived from conformity to a role demanded by a family system or from an identification with another person.

It is often assumed that a sense of identity derives precisely from the very circumstances that are here being described as those which threaten identity—namely, the allocation of a definite role in the family system. But the important difference is that which exists between the recognition of the other person as a unique human being and the recognition of him merely in his role. The difference has been made clear by Buber [1], who writes: 'To be aware of a man, therefore, means in particular to perceive his wholeness as a person determined by the spirit; it means to perceive the dynamic center which stamps his every utterance, action and attitude with the recognizable sign of uniqueness...The perception of one's fellow man as a whole, as a unit, and as unique...is opposed in our time by almost everything that is commonly understood as specifically modern.'[8]

The other way in which a sense of identity is often presumed to arise, namely from identification with a parent figure, presents similar difficulties; the only way in which a true sense of identity can be established is not by an identification in which the child feels he exists only by or through his parent and in which he usurps his parents' role, but by the assimilation on to the original self-schema of the environmental features (primarily the parents) which are suitable, rather as a plant will select from the medium those elements that it requires. It needs to be explained of course where the original schema of the self comes from in the first place. According to Winnicott it arises through the establishment of ego-boundaries by the appropriate physical handling by the mother; this implies that the first sense of identity is that of the biological mother/child unit and that a sense of separate identity arises only if the child's unique (and in the first place innate) needs are recognized by the one person who knows enough to recognize them, the mother, a recognition which shows itself by meeting these needs appropriately. What has been discussed in this chapter is the continuation and extension of this appropriate response to individual needs, in particular as the response concerns the total family configuration rather than the nursing mother alone. The very details of the mother's physical nursing care are affected by the total family pattern, and as the child develops, the influence of the father, the social milieu, and the family structure gain in importance. It is this last factor that is often given insufficient attention; it is becoming increasingly recognized, however, that a sick family is a gestalt, the dynamics of which is important in addition to the individual psychopathology of its members.[9]

The family that has been described in this chapter was sick. It found itself in an unsuitable milieu, adrift from its traditional (and biologically more natural) surroundings, and in a socially inferior position. There resulted a lack of communication with the external world and excessive interdependence of its members, with consequent ambivalence. The insecurity of the family was based not only on its social position but on the husband-wife conflict derived from their differing attitude to the social change. This insecurity caused anxiety over possible disintegration, and a desperate attempt to deny this by the establishment of a family myth of mutual love and loyalty. Just as in time of crises and war the state cannot afford to acknowledge rights of individuality and accepts only rigid role-behaviour orientated towards the welfare of the group, so this family could not allow its individual members to be individuals. The resulting pseudo-mutuality was intolerable to the patient's needs to be recognized as a real person and her illness represented her attempt to escape from the role to which she had been assigned.

References

1. Erikson, Erik H. (1956), 'The Problem of Ego Identity,' *J. Amer. Psychoanal. Assoc.* 4, p. 56.
2. Searles, Harold F. (1959), 'The Effort to Drive the Other Person Crazy: An Element in the Aetiology and Pathology of Schizophrenia.' *Brit J. Med. Psychol.* 32, no. 1.
3. Wynne, L.C., I.M. Rycoff, J. Day, and S.I. Hirsch (1958). 'Pseudo-mutuality in the Family Relations of Schizophrenics,' *Psychiatry* 21, p. 205.
4. Winnicott, D. W. [1954] 1958, 'Metapsychological and Clinical Aspects of Regression within the Psychoanalytic Set-up,' in *Collected Papers*, Tavistock, London.
5. Shaw, George Bernard, (1952), as quoted in Erikson, from *Selected Prose*, Dodd, Mead, New York.
6. Milner, Marion (1955), 'The Role of Illusion in Symbol Formation,' in *New Directions in Psychoanalysis*, edited by Klein, Heimann, and Money-Kyrle. Tavistock, London.
7. Main, T. F. (1957), 'The Ailment,' *Brit. J. Med. Psychol.* 30, p. 129.
8. Buber, Martin (1957), 'Elements of the Interhuman,' *Psychiatry* 20, p. 97.
9. Galdston, Iago, ed. (1958), *The Family in Contemporary Society*, International Universities Press, New York.

3

Passivity and Failure of Identity Formation

Because of an assumption that the natural state of the female is a passive one the problem presented by the symptoms of passivity has been considered, in psychoanalytic literature, as primarily a male one; specifically, the theory centres on the boy's needs to repress his sexual and aggressive drives in the oedipal situation. It is this view that I wish to question here. In the first part of the chapter I shall describe some aspects of the analysis of a man who suffered from passivity, but whose illness and its treatment were in no way out of the ordinary.

Mr. R., a well-built man in his early thirties, suffered from chronic anxiety, inhibitions in his capacity to work, and various somatic symptoms such as headache and fainting attacks. The first serious signs of illness occurred when he was in his early twenties, working in a very junior position in his father's factory; he felt unable to tolerate the discipline which the work demanded, became anxious and developed a backache which incapacitated him for eighteen months. Symptoms had persisted since that time.

The Patient's Early Life and Family Background

Mr. R.'s parents were Jewish emigrants who had begun life in England in lowly circumstances in the East End of London. His father gradually, and with intermittent setbacks, built up a business which was finally very successful, but continued to be haunted by fears of poverty. His philosophy of life centred on work and family security, and he instilled this philosophy into his children, emphasising the sacrifices made for them, their luck compared with his own, and the continual need for vigilance on his part to avoid a return to poverty. However, while thus implying that his children should work as hard as himself, he at the same time needed to show that he was such a successful man that he could supply all their needs without effort on their part. (He became enraged, for instance, when the patient, as a teenager, took a job delivering papers, and later, would boast that everything his son had was his [father's] doing.) Mr. R. described him as an energetic, emotional, insecure man who feigned illness and suffering in order to gain love, and who compensated for his insecurity by the assumption of a godlike infallible wisdom.

His mother, by contrast, was a quiet woman who gave in to her husband's quirks and tantrums, mopping his brow and stroking his head, fetching his slippers and aspirins, and soothing the children whose crying disturbed him.

The patient was the third of four children, having an elder brother and sister and a younger sister. The elder two he regarded as essentially masculine in character, having identified closely with his father. When he was born his mother was said to have declared: 'This one is going to be mine.' His was a painless and easy birth and his infancy continued to be uncommonly trouble free. He was (bottle) fed by his mother and toilet trained early and effectively. 'You are not like the others,' his mother would say to him, 'You are like me.' His elder sister had wanted him to be a girl. However, she took a great interest in him and the two were always together. In their games she always took the boy's role and he the girl's.

His father, too, regarded him as feminine, and although this was probably to some extent an acceptance of the situation described above, he had reasons of his own for so doing. He himself was the elder of two sons, and his own father had treated them quite differently, regarding him as tough and masculine and giving him beatings, and his brother as feminine, soft, and loveable. It appeared that this problem was repeated for the patient who, in complete contrast to his brother, received no beatings; and in later life his father would say to him, 'You could never do the job Bob does.'

It is little surprising therefore that the patient grew to be the delicate and sensitive one of the family, fainting at the sight of blood, losing his fights in spite of superior strength (for he was physically well-built) and placing great reliance on the support and drive of his mother and sister. He accepted his mother's perception of the marriage as one in which a hard and selfish, unfaithful and insensitive taskmaster imposed his will on a long-suffering wife—a view which was perhaps all the more convincing in that his mother probably contrived to perpetuate this kind of relationship for masochistic purposes. (That there was possibly another side to the story, the patient learnt in adult life from his father, who told him that the mother was sexually unresponsive to him, causing him to seek satisfaction elsewhere.)

Reflecting on these events during analysis, Mr. R.'s complaint about his childhood situation was not only that his masculinity had been stamped on, but that he had not been genuinely loved, that he had been used by his mother to fulfil her expectations of an ideal child entirely her own, by his sister to support her masculine strivings, and by his father as a foil to his godlike pronouncements.

The oppression which he felt in this situation is suggested by his memory of a recurrent nightmare during which he would feel 'smothered by a great cloud.' His chief escape from the conflict brought about by the suppression of his natural impulses was by fantasy and masturbation, often of an omnipotent nature. One recurring theme was that he would rescue a poor, starved boy and give him food and riches. Many times he would imagine he was a girl, dressing up as one or pushing his penis out of sight between his legs.

The Patient's Adult Life

His first employment was with his father; but at this time he began to show signs of adolescent rebellion towards his family, came to resent his father's bossing him about, and eventually left. His subsequent jobs were (probably through unconscious design) catastrophic failures, however, and he returned to his father—as he had always known he would—pleading to be re-installed. His father, with a show of reluctance, accepted him again and it was soon after this that his symptoms began.

His masculine inhibitions and his excessive indulgence in fantasy of an exhibitionistic-voyeuristic nature did not prevent the development of an apparently normal physical sexual functioning. He was terrified of getting married, but did so, surprisingly, to a non-Jew, against the opposition of his family, and to someone who was in many ways the antithesis of his mother, a matter-of-fact, secure, undemonstrative woman who remained relatively immune to the hysterical manoeuvres which had been effective in getting his mother to spoil him. It seemed like an attempt to jump out of the fantasy system of his family and go his own way. Although his wife's placidity drove him to distraction at times, and although he behaved to her with alternating extremes of sadism and masochism, his marriage had remained fairly stable, and there appeared to be genuine feeling on both sides. He had a daughter two-and-a-half-years old. The birth of his twin boys, just before his coming to see me, had increased his chronic anxiety almost to the breaking point. Not only did he feel resentful jealousy towards his wife, whose maternal love for the boys he equated with his own mother's possessive love for him, but he was unable to touch them.

The Patient's Present Life

The patient was caught in a net in his working life. He could not leave his father's firm because he was convinced that on his own he was unemployable and would starve—a belief which his father fostered and encouraged—and, as he gradually realised, he feared that his father's morale, which rested on the utter dependence of his sons, would collapse if he showed his capacity to leave. Work within the factory was intolerable to him because, although he showed ability, both his father and brother either took over or took credit for his work and he would be unable to stand up for himself. With increasing frequency there would be ferocious scenes in which he would shout and curse and walk out of the building, only to capitulate in the end. It became clear how he arranged these scenes, enjoyed the drama and display, identified himself with a sensitive woman, and needed the final surrender. Fantasies of castration pervaded his thoughts and sometimes included a passive (physical) homosexual surrender to his father. It became possible to relate these occurrences to the family problem described above and his need to fit in with it, to reveal the masochistic gratifications involved, the repressed revenge fantasies, which were to some extent enacted in surreptitious attacks on his father's and brother's schemes, the oedipal fantasies involved in a situation in which the three men fought for possession of the symbolic mother (the factory) and furthermore, to relate some of this to the transference. As a result of his increased insight (and, it must be added, to a magic introjection of my analytic potency) he became more assertive in his work, and started to stand up for himself. The results were interesting. His brother became manifestly less sure of himself and succumbed to illness, after which Mr. R. welcomed him back with a patronising solicitude 'as though he were a woman.' On the day after he had given his father a dressing down, his father, too, retired hurt and took to his bed, whereupon the patient felt terribly guilty and became preoccupied with worry about his tonsils, looking at them in a mirror 'at least fifty times' during the evening.

His passivity at work depended on a number of factors: inhibitions of his sexual rivalry towards father and brother, deference to his father's omniscience, angry and self-protective withdrawal from situations in which his efforts were patronised or discouraged, and a guilt which derived from his aggressive feelings and his sulky withdrawal of interest in the business.

On the other hand, his activity at work—and, in relation to his subordinate, he was often extremely active—depended on a magic identification with his father and had a spurious quality to it. He would swear and shout like his father, with the same intonations, and was compulsively addicted to using the same techniques of bullying. In his dreams about his employees, he committed a similar homosexual rape of them as he, in fantasy, experienced from his father. (It is interesting to note, in connection with the similarity of voice—a deep, masculine one—that both he and his father suffered from a phobia of laryngeal cancer.)

His domestic life took a rather similar turn, during the early stages of analysis, as his work relationships. At the start of analysis he was unassertive in the home and left things, in a sulky way, to his wife. 'Why should I do things in *your* house?' he would complain. In sexual intercourse with his wife—although there was no obvious disorder of physical function—he derived little satisfaction and felt that his penis was swallowed up by her. His increasing assertiveness towards her often took on arrogant form and was followed by self-abasement, usually in a way that symbolised castration.

His Behaviour during Analysis

Mr. R. was a friendly and likeable man who, despite his manifold defensive attempts to escape a real object-relation and replace it by a controlled and artificial one, remained basically a warm person.

At the beginning he treated me with the utmost respect, addressing me as 'Sir,' taking my superiority for granted, and regarding himself as an unworthy nuisance lucky to command my attention. Not only was he never late, but he was never early, preferring to sit outside in his car rather than risk causing me any possible inconvenience by untimely arrival. He never used the lavatory. On the couch he behaved in a less inhibited way, but admitted, on questioning, his awareness that such behaviour was expected by psychoanalysts, and his need to conform to this.

This type of behaviour represented a masochistic denigration of himself coupled with repression of his urges (both constructive and destructive) and a compensatory idealisation of me to whom he could then turn for inspiration, strength and help. He hung on to my words as though they were magic charms, encouraging me at the end of each session to make a succinct formulation that would last him the rest of the day. In one session he told me how beautifully arranged were the flowers in my consulting room and how he would like to paint them. Later in the session he reported a dream: a woman gave him some homemade rhubarb wine. It did not taste particularly good to him but, in order to please her, he told her it did. I suggested that his reaction in the dream applied also to his valuation of what I gave him in analysis and also, as a child, what his mother gave him. In the next session he commented, without any intervening analysis on my part, that the flowers were not perhaps so out of the ordinary as he had imagined and were not after all very suitable for painting.

Another feature of his relationship to me seems at first sight to contradict the behaviour hitherto described. He regarded himself as having special importance in my eyes. Although reasonably well aware that it was a matter of chance and convenience that caused me to see him at my own home rather than at my consulting room in town, he continued to see in this signs of special love and privilege. Moreover, his analysis would be unique. He believed (with undue optimism) that it would be the quickest on record; and when he began to doubt this he came to hope that out of it would develop a new technique that would be 'as great an advance on psychoanalysis as psychoanalysis was on hypnotism.' However, certain other features of these wishes suggested that it would not be all gain. The chief claim for being treated as special lay in his delicateness and vulnerability. Just as his mother had been solicitous about his physical health, so I should be about his mental condition, and on this score was most aggrieved and reproachful if I made any but the softest of interpretations. Furthermore this spoiling of him brought with it the penalty of having to be sufficiently nice and docile to warrant it. Once when the shouting of my children impinged unduly on the session and passed without comment from him, I asked him why. He admitted that the thought had occurred to him, 'Why don't you keep your kids quiet?', but said that he considered he had no right to make such demands as I already treated him with special consideration, seeing him at my home, and so forth. The idea that he was special, although to some extent equated with omnipotent overvaluation, was not only compensation involving denial of his impotence and hatred, but the acceptance of a role, similar to the one enforced on him in childhood, in which his importance resided only in being passive in the face of another's (his mother's) omnipotent and possessive fantasies.

His resentment at my (supposedly) casting him in the role of my special and delicate prodigy emerged on occasions when he would declare that I had no interest in him. Once, when I asked him where he supposed my interest lay, he immediately answered, 'Psychoanalysis,' a remark which I interpreted as a transference from his belief that his mother was interested in being a mother rather than in him.

He believed that I planned and could forecast his every move, that I had him in complete control like a puppet. Bitterly resenting this situation and feeling as helpless against it as he had felt in childhood, he derived as much satisfaction from it as he could and fostered it wherever possible. His emotional behaviour was far from being as spontaneous as it appeared, and was largely an act on his part, designed to arouse my attention, pity, and love. This attempt to live through the other person gave rise to an inordinate degree of self-consciousness, partly because it required eternal vigilance to maintain such a controlled relationship, and partly as a result of identifying himself with the observer. He was almost never able to stop observing himself, planning his behaviour, and calculating its effect on me, and his compulsion to act in this way was a torment to him.

Mr. R.'s resentment at being deprived of spontaneous action caused him to attempt to control me not only for the reasons already given but as an aggressive measure of revenge. He tried to make me self-conscious, too, and to paralyse my moves, feeding me with questions to which he already knew the answers and could forecast mine with some accuracy, and gaining satisfaction from my forecast silence when I ceased to respond to his spurious questions. Projection of his own controlling urges onto me increased the intensity of this vicious circle. Much of the time he adopted a playful and bantering quality of tone, thereby detaching himself from the experience, escaping from my perception, and confusing me. Sometimes, after making a remark, he would add, 'Don't kid yourself. I didn't mean it. I only said it to get your reaction.' His elusiveness was coupled with the possession of a secret self—which he was aware of and could describe vividly—and which remained safe and untouchable, observing me with detached irony, in the way he had preserved himself from his family's intrusive policies as a child.

Further aggression was relieved by the masochistic way in which he sometimes brought his problems to me, passively awaiting the solution, holding me entirely responsible for the success of the session. The denied aggression behind these techniques returned, however, in the unpleasant form of a fierce Alsatian dog which he often imagined would be awaiting him on my doorstep. The real and spontaneous behaviour, of which he was terrified, would sometimes break through, following analysis of his control, in the form of a kind of fit. During these episodes his head would shake from side to side, he would sweat and groan and say such things as, 'I'm frightened. I wish you would hold me.' 'I'm not here. There's no me.' Although these 'fits' contained a noticeable charge of self-display, my overall impression of him at these moments was of a genuinely frightened, helpless child who had lost his bearings, and it was to this element that I felt most called on to respond, suggesting to him that he had allowed himself to give up his need for control and to trust in the spontaneous relationship.

In an attempt to relieve his feeling of emptiness he undertook, in a confused way, two operations which were diametrically opposed in character: an undefended attempt to be receptive towards the real nature of things and, superimposed upon this, a passive and exhibitionistic homosexual wish to be penetrated by a magic penis. I felt that the abandonment of defensive control and the emergence of something felt to be not himself was essentially of the same nature as, although of less intensity than, what Winnicott[1] describes as occurring in the analyses of some schizoid patients, and which he refers to as a 'regression to the real self'. The blankness of the experience suggests that it may possess a significance like that of the dream screen, of which Rycroft writes:

> Dreams showing the dream screen are likely to occur when patients with narcissistic fixations are attempting to re-establish emotional contact with the external world.[2]

That is, (to use Winnicott's terminology) at times when defensive control is given up and the 'real self' allowed to emerge and seek out objects.

The gradual diminution of intensity of these attacks during analysis was accompanied by a re-orientation towards the world and to myself. He recognised that hitherto he had regarded the world 'as though it were made by my father': fixed, rigid, unresponsive, and entirely known, with no differentiation between organic and inorganic matter. Now, with a mixture of surprise, hope, and apprehension, he saw that there was possibly an altogether different view of it, one that included mystery, unpredictability, and insecurity.

In a similar way he suffered a gradual disillusionment in me. His previous idealisation of me, although it contained a static deadness, ('You live in a different world from me,' he would complain, 'I am surrounded by a concrete wall with the real me inside, thinking the whole business is phony') was something he gave up only with difficulty. It involved, too, the giving up of the magic use to which he put analysis, as is suggested by the following dream:

He was pale and drawn and had something wrong with his eye. (It is interesting that this dream preceded an attack of migraine.) He went to a man who knew how to help such cases, but this man himself suffered from similar problems. The scene changed, and, he coughed up, from the regions of his tonsils, a bottle marked 'Nerve Tone,' which had been there a long time and had worn thin. After recounting this dream he remarked, 'I wish you were a wizard. I used to think you were.' 'Nerve Tone' immediately brought to mind 'psychoanalysis.' The dream suggests that the introjection of my magic potency which had previously counterbalanced his impotence and inadequacy had 'worn thin' and needed to be expelled, but with reluctance.

The Analysis of His 'God-Complex'

On one occasion he started the session as follows: 'Last night I felt so ill. I told my wife I was ill. My skin felt horrible and I was weak and I kept looking to see if there were ulcers on my tonsils. I have a dream to tell you. There was a big ugly tough Russian woman with a square head. She has just bought a house for retiring—L-shaped—and she seemed to turn it inside out and it became more valuable, like that chap, everything he touches turns to gold. She was strong, seemed to be in command of everything.'

I asked him to describe this turning inside out. 'It's like an orange with a slit in it,' he replied, 'You turn it inside out and the good thing comes out. I know! It was like a vagina and the thing inside was a penis. That's because she's masculine.'

Asked about his associations to buying a house, he replied: 'My mother's buying houses now; she's taken over from the old man (his father) and runs that side of the business. She runs him more and more. When he retires she'll run him altogether. He's terrified of retiring, thinks he'll die.'

I pointed out how that dream fit in with this picture of his mother swallowing his father now and how he had always described his father as being the one who had the knack of turning things into gold. He seemed to be changing his mind about who was the strong one. 'Yes,' he said, 'I feel sorry for my father now. My mother's really the power and he's sick.'

I suggested that he was preoccupied with the problem as to whom to identify with if his father was no longer God. He was afraid he would have to turn to his mother and be feminine. But even then he was still looking for the idealised magic penis (the gold) in her possession. What he couldn't risk was to give up the magic and see them as ordinary people.

'My father'd die if he was ordinary,' he said. 'It's not just my imagination. Nearly every day now he says "You don't want me here. I'm no use (to the factory) any longer, am I?" And he cries when he talks of retiring. He's got to be God or nothing. How can I take his place when he's like that? I wish my parents were happy people.'

We discussed the question of the objective truth about his father's feelings. I suggested that although the belief that his father would collapse if he gave up being God to his son probably existed in his father's mind also. Although the father would not *necessarily* collapse if he retired, the patient had the added problem of his *own* need to support this God illusion. 'That's probably true,' he said, 'He'd find something else to boost himself up with. But what about me? I'd collapse without this God thing. Who can I identify with? I can't identify with you. You're feminine!' I asked him why he thought me feminine. 'You're not a Jew,' he said, 'that's tied up with this God.' I said that I thought that because I was not a Jew I was ordinary and that meant I could only help him to be ordinary, which to him was a frightening prospect. 'Ordinary people don' t count with my family,' he said, 'You've got to be a genius.'

In the following session he again reverted to preoccupation with his tonsils. I drew his attention to the similarity between the thing-inside-the-mouth and the penis-inside-the-vagina of the dream, and his idealisation of the latter and fear of the former's destructive potency. 'Yes, I think it's cancer,' he said. It seemed to me that his fear of cancer derived, firstly, from the belief that dependence for identity on his internalised and idealised father-image threatened to eat up his real identity and destroy the proper experience of life; and secondly, from it's symbolisation of his own denied and projected aggression concealed in the idealised image.

A few days later he again referred to the dream. He was feeling somewhat depersonalised and commented that some of the things in the consulting room were standing out and appearing excessively solid. He agreed with my interpretation that they represented his projected self-penis concealed from ordinary vision and said :'It's like the hidden thing in the peeled orange, in the dream. I don't get into the vagina from outside. I'm already inside.' It would seem that the idealised image of the parental penis contained the projected image of his own real penis. The usual place for its concealment, however, was in the image of a young girl—a phenomenon he described later.

This internal gold symbolised not only his parents' magic power, his own masculinity, but the individuality which he preserved from his family's attempt to mould him to an alien pattern. It has already been described how he kept a secret, inviolable self safe from the wishes of his parents to whom, on the surface, he was extremely placatory and malleable. On one occasion he said to me: 'I used to keep my secret self inside my mouth. It was my tonsils.' But this secret self, although it contained the basis of his true individuality, had become estranged from reality, idealised, and fused with the alien and idealised image of his parents.

One factor which was important in helping him to emerge from his God-complex was the analysis of those elements which deprived him of a normal and healthy relationship with his father. Not least among those factors was a divided family system in which he and his mother were in a 'separate camp' from his father. He gradually came to realise the degree to which his own low estimation of his father mirrored that of his mother and derived from it. His mother's seduction of him and deception of his father (talking contemptuously behind his back, etc.) put him in the position of believing that either his father was not worthy of honest dealing or that his mother was a cheat. Furthermore, in this context, the concept of shared love was an alien one. Of the alternatives he chose to believe in his mother and accept her estimation of the situation. This choice not only affected his estimation of his father but probably affected his father's real behaviour. The absence of real interchange between father and son, of physical intimacy and shared ideology, was replaced by secret idealistic identifications with his omniscience, preoccupation with fantasies of anal incorporation, and displacement of his father's potency onto his mother and sister. At the point at which insight was gained into the yearning for his father, obscured by these mechanisms and its reappearance in the transference, he said: 'The analysis has really started now.'

The Patient's Relationship with His Mother

Although, according to the family myth, the sole possessor of power and value was the father, the patient nevertheless feared his mother and, as the dream reported in the previous section shows, regarded her as powerful also. This was partly because he saw through the myth—in a dissociated way—and recognised that in fact his mother did have power in the household, and partly because he conceived her to possess power, or liable to possess power, vicariously.

'I've always felt I shouldn't have a body,' he said on one occasion. 'My mother didn't like it. She didn't like my penis. I suppose she didn't like men. Felt badly done by them. It sounds silly, I know, but I have always felt like saying to her: "You have it. I'll give it you as a present."'

Elaborating on his relationship with his daughter, he added: 'I am to her as my mother is to me. She is part of me.' He agreed with my suggestion that his daughter symbolised his penis, and expressed his fear that it was his possessive and parasitic attitude towards her that made her so meek and passive. These thoughts stimulated memories of his mother's embarrassment at handling his penis, of her reluctance to deal with him directly as a person (by understanding) or as a physical being (by bodily contact), preferring to leave him to the care of a nursemaid. He was perplexed by the apparent contrast between this attitude of hers and her anxious and possessive concern for him. It seemed to me, however, that his description of his mother was entirely consistent with that of a mother who compensates for a failure to make genuine contact with her child by an attitude of anxious overprotection.

His Exhibitionism and Scopophilia

Many of Mr. R.'s dreams were exhibitionistic in character—a typical one, early in analysis, depicted his being exhibited at Olympia as an example of what analysis can do; and during the sessions he was very preoccupied with my awareness and estimation of his appearance and performance. He recalled how as a child he used to exhibit his buttocks at the window, and gaze at himself in the mirror, sometimes displaying his genitals, at other times concealing them and imagining himself to be a girl (presumably when anxieties over phallic display proved intolerable). This need to display himself sexually, either to himself or to others, persisted into adult life, and his central fantasy was the typical one of display before a young girl.

During one session he described how he had been shopping and felt utterly alone, lost and disintegrated as soon as he was away from his car but felt better after he had summoned the courage to enter a restaurant and have a meal. This experience seemed to me to represent the feelings of a child, who had never learnt to function on his own but had to rely on others to 'carry' him or on something magic inside or outside as a substitute. He went on to describe how later in the day he met a young girl whom he tried to impress and about whom he had fantasies of seduction and self-display. It seemed that he was attempting to compensate for his previous feelings of nothingness but that again he was depending on something external to himself (the girl's admiration).

His fantasies of seducing or displaying himself before a young girl could be seen to derive from a need to reverse the original situation with his mother and sister, in which he had been the small and helpless one, lost in admiration for them. They—his memory was of his sister in particular—were the big strong ones, the source of life and activity, and he lived vicariously through them. Now he could not stand tall women, and if he was attracted to an adult woman she was usually very small (his wife was an exception to this). He agreed with my interpretation that the small girl represented a penis and that he now possessed, in the girl, a penis, just as, he believed, there was a mutual fantasy that he had been the penis of his mother and sister.

Fenichel[3] in discussing problems of transvestism and exhibitionism, comments not only on the importance of the equation phallus=girl, but adds that the clown is a further equivalent, a contention which is borne out by the study of the patient under discussion who was the joker of the family and who had continued into adult life to rely on his capacity for buffoonery to establish himself socially. Fenichel points out that the transvestite and the clown have the advantage of being able to display a concealed phallus or one that will not be taken seriously. It would seem that the concealment lies in the presentation of the opposite of reality, masculinity being replaced by femininity, and seriousness by ridiculousness, so that, as in a detective story, the concealed item is to be found in the least likely place. Mr. R. took a special delight in such situations and on occasions would deceive people and flourish the deception under their noses, sometimes knowing that they were aware of the deception but not in a position to unmask it. This latter finesse was of particular value to him: not only was a more flagrant display of the real situation possible but there were added delights involved in the excitement of risk and the triumph over others who themselves could be made to appear and feel ridiculous.

Mr. R.'s exhibitionistic fantasies and manoeuvres, although active insofar as they manifested an urge to reveal his existence, contained markedly passive elements. Because the source of strength lay in the girl's youth, spontaneous naïveté and phallic symbolism, he was a passive recipient of these qualities, and because the fantasy contained a large element of self-display, she, his object, was the one who evaluated him and bestowed identity. Thus, owing to his failure to exist as a subject in command of his own impulses, he secondarily sought to be the object of another with whom he was identified or even to be (as when looking in a mirror) his own object.

Scopophilia had an importance in Mr. R.'s life equal to that of his exhibitionism. He watched bedroom windows, sometimes with the aid of binoculars, hoping for a glimpse of a woman undressing, and sometimes followed girls in the street weaving fantasies of seduction around them, but stopping short of any action. Unfamiliarity, secrecy, and control were important elements in these preoccupations.

By contrast, when he came to see me he behaved as though he were in blinkers, although his intense and guilty interest in the rest of the house, my family, and myself gradually emerged. Sometimes his interest in my wife was projected, as, for instance, when he had an urgent desire to look at the windows of the house opposite in the hope of seeing a woman undressing. That this scopophilic tendency had its origin in childhood is suggested by his memory of frequently peering through his elder sister's bedroom in order to watch her undressing.

Mr. R. had a keen and expert interest in photography, a hobby which he sometimes considered taking up professionally, and one which well served his scopophilic impulses. On occasions he took pictures of girls in bathing costumes on the beach, unbeknownst to them, and had also photographed his own genitals in the mirror. One day he came to the session enraged because his wife, without his knowledge or permission, had invited a professional photographer to the house to take shots of the children. Not only did he feel slighted by his wife's obvious belief in the superior technical ability of the professional man but he was tormented by the fantasy that the photographer had seduced her. He felt particularly impotent towards a man who supposedly used his own methods of secret (symbolic) seduction and possession.

Scopophilia was a useful defence against Mr. R.'s active (notably sexual) wishes. Hypercathexis of one particular mode of sensual experience replaced a feared relationship of total experience with the object in which all modes would be appropriately used. There was further advantage in the use of the visual mode in that, firstly, attention was thereby drawn away from the genital zone, and secondly, engagement of the object could take place at considerable physical distance (especially with the aid of binoculars) and secrecy was thereby greatly facilitated. The secretness of the operation in turn was conducive to the development of fantasies surrounding it, and therefore an idealised and controlled experience could be substituted for a real, overt, testable one with all its concomitant risks.

Perception is ordinarily an active process, a preliminary to and contribution towards full engagement of the object. The type of perception involved in scopophilia is, by contrast, passive. Mr. R. did not perceive his objects as part of a process of real engagement of them, but in such a way as to enable him to derive narcissistic gain by his association with something possessing ideal value. He either entered into them, into their chamber, their lives, and partook of their spontaneity in unseen conditions (stole his way into them in secret) or he forcibly introjected them into his own world (again in secret) as for instance by taking photographs of them. What was valued by him was never the people themselves. His interest lay in their bodies or parts of their bodies which he imbued with magic significance, just as he did certain items in other spheres: food, racial characteristics, social status, odd bits of knowledge, and money. Since potency resided in these items he himself was passive towards them; he could possess them and even exhibit them, but they were never intrinsic to him. And the people to whom he related remained valueless except insofar as they themselves happened to be associated with such special items.

It can be seen from this that for Mr. R. exhibitionism and scopophilia—though potentially a source of normal activity and perception*—were essentially passive in nature. In both there was an addiction to idealised objects which served as sources of potency by magical introjection or projection, but were inimical to the sharing and communication that characterises active and realistic relationships.

The Outcome of the Analysis

This chapter is concerned with the causes and nature of passivity and not with its attempted cure, but perhaps I have given sufficient material to provoke some interest in this patient, and I will very briefly recount the ending of treatment.

His analysis lasted four years. Shortly before it ended he went and had his tonsils out. This was an ordeal for him, as he had been preoccupied with the question of the operation for years as it had a rich symbolic meaning, but he finally met it with courage. It seems to me that two opposite fantasies, both of which centred on the idea of initiation, were especially significant: (1) the sacrifice to the father in order that he would be allowed adult status; and (2) the renunciation of an

---

*The pathological hypercathexis of perception constituted by scopophilia had its counterpart in a creative talent for painting. Mr. R. had retained some of the naïve vision characteristic of the artist.

alien, idealised, internal phallus in order to pave the way for the development of an identity more real. The first I regarded as neurotic; the second, realistic.

At the end of analysis he still remained capable of a disquieting amount of anxiety in situations which required him to exhibit himself in public, but he could now assert his rights. He and his brother together were successful in managing the factory without the aid of their father. Sexuality was no longer a mere physical instinct to be satisfied and he came to feel it as intimately connected with the whole of his personality.

But what, to my mind, was of most significance was a change in his basic feeling about the world and his relations to it, a change that was epitomised by his comment, quoted above, that he had previously felt the world to be rigid and entirely known; it now became more alive and so did he. This change could be conceptualised in many ways, one of which is that of a transformation from a passive to an active mode of existence.

Conclusions about the Origin and Manifestations of the Patient's Passivity

Mr. R. was born into a family which, insofar as his memories and the reconstructions in analysis are correct, far from awaiting his arrival with impartial expectancy, had preconceived ideas about the role he should fulfil. He was the one who, at last, was to be his mother's own possession; he was to be a little girl for his sister to play with; and there were some indications that, for his father, he was to fill the role of the younger, feminine brother. To these particular requirements have to be added those deriving from the norms of the culture into which he was born, for instance, that he be able to control his eliminatory functions within the first year of life.

Several elements in this situation predispose towards the tendency on his part to accept the passive position:

1. Insofar as the family wished for and tried to produce the child required of them rather than accept a child who would develop according to his potentialities, he was expected to be passive and inert. This prime expectation of passivity underlies and subsumes the other factors.

2. He was regarded by his mother and sister as an object of their possession (in fantasy, a bodily appendage) who would not stray from them but exist through them and in order to enhance their own self-esteem.

3. He was estranged from his own body, not only because body and identity are intrinsically related, but because of the attitude towards his body taken by his mother in her physical handling of him.

4. He was deprived of his sexual identity, thereby becoming estranged from a fundamental biological mode of active engagement with the object.

5. Because the sexual identity of which he was deprived was male, he was also prevented from the more overt expression of activity that is characteristic of the male—deriving not only from the biological function but social sanction in areas that are not clearly biological. (It is doubtful whether a male deprived of his masculinity is essentially made more passive—in the sense in which this term is developed later in the chapter—than a woman deprived of her femininity, but he certainly appears so, and from a social point of view, is so; and the shame he experiences is greater.)

6. He was cut off from the meaningful relationship with his father necessary for the development of a masculine identity, in place of which he was presented with a spurious male identity personified by his father, whose image he could only incorporate as an alien thing in his psyche.

7. He was cut off from meaningful relationships not only within the family but outside it. As his father's and mother's special son, he acted outside the household not as himself but as his family's agent, and could not therefore actively participate with ordinary people as an equal (particularly not with those who were not of his parents' race). In other words, he lived by and through his parents' self-idealisation.

Hitherto the question of the patient's own contribution to his passivity has not been considered. Assuming—and there is no evidence to the contrary—that he was born healthy, it would consist of his acceptance, as a necessary measure, of the situation in which he found himself, and of the way in which such behaviour became useful to him as a defensive manoeuvre and brought secondary gain.

These factors can be considered under the following headings:

1. He came to believe—and, apparently, with some justification—that passivity was necessary in order to gain the love and acceptance of his family and to acquire a recognisable and relatively stable identity.

2. The hate engendered in him by deprivation of real identity could be expressed by a sulky and negative attitude to life.

3. The pain consequent upon a failure of response to his active strivings to relate was avoided by withdrawing from real relationships.

4. Passivity enabled him to conceal his strong aggressive impulses and served as a masochistic defence against guilt feelings.

5. His passivity enabled him not only to avoid the difficulties and dangers which accompany participation and growth but to gain the special attentions and privileges which, particularly in our culture, are allotted to women, children, and the sick, insofar as they manifest passivity (incapacity). This gain served as a defence against feelings of envy, hate, and the guilt engendered thereby.

6. Failure of autonomous functioning led to a greedy, passive, and parasitic desire to extract the good which inhabited the object—('I want to suck individuality out of you,' he once said)—and denial of this greed resulted in further passivity in the form of pathological generosity and self-denial.

The manifestations of his passivity are in many cases inherent in the origins, but a summary of them would include the following points:

1. He lacked real identity, and attempted to compensate for this by reliance on a magic identity extraneous to himself (readily available

owing to his parents' self-idealisation), involving the use of projection, introjection, splitting, and denial. He could at the same time feel superlatively potent and yet deny that the potency was really his.

2. His exhibitionism, while giving the impression of activity and temporarily enhancing his self-esteem, really served passive aims, for he performed for and depended on the valuation of the object whom he idealised and with whom he was identified. Particularly insofar as he represented the object's performing penis he was a mere appendage.

3. Similarly his scopophilia was passive in that he entered secretly into the life of another and lived through them.

4. His exhibitionism, scopophilia, and the accompanying fantasy life constituted a withdrawal from direct, real, and active engagement of the object.

5. His homosexual wishes were associated with the adoption of a feminine identity and the desire to be penetrated and fertilised by the idealised penis. This was a passive manoeuvre in that it was the adoption of a biologically alien identity; his passive anal incorporative aims had little to do with genuinely receptive vaginal ones.

6. Spontaneous and creative action was replaced by controlling behaviour, the essential aim of which was to prevent change.

What I have tried to convey in the first part of this chapter is the way in which, during the analysis of this patient, I found convincing the idea that his passivity was a consequence of having been placed in a passive position in which identity growth was unavailable to him. I recognise that the picture I have given of his childhood is a hypothetical reconstruction for which I have no corroborative evidence, but I hope to show in what follows that it at least has a logical consistency.

Discussion

Classical psychoanalytical theory postulates that male passivity constitutes a retreat from the feared consequences of active, phallic strivings in the oedipal situation; that the son adopts a passive attitude towards his father by the adoption of a feminine or infantile role which he is unable to relinquish.

Although this formulation has proved useful in clinical practise it is based on ideas that have questionable validity: that the natural state of the infant is passive; that the natural state of the woman is passive; that the terms 'activity' or 'action' can be restrictively used, without distortion of reality, to denote specific modes of behaviour (e.g., phallic) characteristic of certain classes of person (e.g., males). In pursuing this question I am relying on the belief that current usage of these terms is not a minor matter of verbal taste but betrays significant and erroneous assumptions about persons and their development.

Infantile Action

It is one of the findings—perhaps the most dramatic finding—of psychoanalysis that there is more to a child than had hitherto been suspected, that his life is richer, that he is more of a person, that he is more capable of feeling, thought, and action than had been accredited to him by his elders and betters. Yet on this issue, surprisingly, Freud's position is paradoxical. Although the protagonist of the movement which has emancipated the child, he underestimates, in his theoretical formulations, the child's capacity for action. A lucid argument against these formulations was made by Schachtel:

> Freud saw the ontogenetic beginnings of man as dominated completely by the pleasure principle, and his concept of this principle is such that it represents essentially a flight from or a fight against life and reality: it is the quest to return to a state without stimulation, excitation, tension, and striving....
>
> What Freud overlooked was that from birth on the infant and child also shows an eagerness to turn towards an increasing variety of things in the environing reality and that the sensory contact with them is enjoyed rather than experienced as disturbing excitation. While at first this is true of only relatively few, impinging stimuli, already in the first weeks the infant tries to seek them out or to recover them if they are lost. Most of these encounters are sought not in order to abolish the stimuli or the excitation caused by them, and increasingly not in order to still hunger or thirst or as a detour on the way to return to the comfort of sleep, but out of a growing urge to get in touch with and explore the world around the infant.[4]

Schachtel adds substance to his views by a detailed analysis of affect, perception, and attention. He believes that in addition to affects which have the function of ridding the organism of excessive drive-tension, there exist 'activity-affects.' He writes:

> While the hungry infant's restlessness and crying is the most dramatic instance of its emotional behaviour, we can observe other instances which show a different kind of emotional behaviour from the first or second day of the infant's life on. When we watch the sucking behaviour of infants in nursing we can see in quite a few of them an attitude which shows all the signs of eager concentration. Here the picture is entirely different from the restless behaviour. The torso and the limbs are held quite still, and the whole energy is concentrated on the sucking activity. This activity itself is the eagerly pursued and gratifying goal of the infant.

(A revision of affect-theory on these lines would similarly seem to be required by Rycroft's [1963] view of the nature of the primary and secondary process.)

The further one goes back ontogenetically the less does the child's behaviour seem like action, but one has also to take into account the fact that, since his powers of communicating to us become less and his activity increasingly different from ours and strange to us, the more we are likely to consider it alien and lacking in the quality of action. Schachtel's description of the infant's interest in his environment, and his capacity to focus his activity suggest that, even at the start of his life he is more integrated, more of a psychological being, more of a person, and less of a reflex mechanism than we have hitherto recognised. Certainly he is so regarded by his mother, who is the only person really attuned to his communications and who is likely to have an intuitively correct perception of him.[5]

Feminine Action

The erroneous attribution of passivity is liable to be made about the woman not only because of her inferior social position consequent upon the superior physical strength of the male, but because her natural mode of functioning is very unlike that of the man and does not manifest itself in an immediate and striking way.

Freud—as has been pointed out by several writers, most of whom are outside the main trend of the psychoanalytic movement—was not himself free from this bias. Despite the improved status given to feminine psychology by the work of some psychoanalysts, notably Melanie Klein, the equation is still made between femininity and passivity, to the detriment of theory. An exceptional criticism was made by Hermann in 1934.[6] Deploring the fact that 'in psychoanalytic literature we often find "masculine" equated with "activity,"' he wrote:

It is possible that there are certain preconceptions which do violence to the facts and cause these general terms to be used in a restricted or garbled sense. For instance, 'activity' is taken to denote a *special* mode of activity while the fact that there is *another kind of activity* in the female (as evidenced, e.g., in coquetry and seduction), that is not even repressed or denied, is nevertheless ignored.

It is perhaps debatable to what extent Hermann's example of feminine activity—coquetry—is of an intrinsic or socially conditioned quality. Certainly, better examples could have been chosen.

The woman who accepts this view of herself is obliged, in her efforts to acquire status, either to emulate the man—in reality or fantasy—or to idealise the state of passivity; to become either a 'phallic' woman or a masochistic one. Insofar as she chooses the latter course she can feel morally superior to the man who becomes, in her eyes, a selfish unfeeling beast with dirty sexual wishes; she may make him feel ashamed of himself; and she may steer the whole pattern of life into passivity and stasis; but her victory is a hollow one.

Possible Reasons for Mistaken Attributions of Passivity

Apparent, as opposed to real, passivity exists when a person is pursuing his aim in the most appropriate manner yet, to the observer (and perhaps to himself), his behaviour appears to be passive in character. The reason for such a misapprehension may lie in the confusing manner of his behaviour or in the bias of the observer. The former condition applies when the action does not manifest itself immediately and blatantly since it involves the use of complex techniques and periods of quiescence and/or it centres on releasing or developing the action of another person. The latter condition applies when the observer, either because he equates action in general with his own peculiar brand of it, or, for any other reason, fails to perceive the real nature and aims of the person under observation.

Criteria of behaviour are usually established by those in power and types of functioning which do not measure up to such criteria are considered inadequate, wrong, unhealthy, or lacking in action. Qualification for membership of the elite power group is variable but in most societies (up to, if not including, contemporary Western society) there are at least four categories of persons who are excluded from this group: women, children, the mentally sick, and criminals. The situation is complicated, however, by the fact that the disinherited group adopt measures to regain power which rely less on a direct challenge of the myth of the superiority of the power group than upon an acceptance and exploitation of it. Although this manoeuvre may constitute of a real challenge to power, it necessarily involves a sacrifice of identity and the taking up of a fundamentally parasitic position. This state of affairs makes difficult any attempt to assess the validity of the various attributions made about these groups—that they are passive, inadequate, and so forth—since it becomes necessary to distinguish between real intrinsic qualities and those self-portrayed as a manoeuvre during the course of a battle for power. The fact, therefore, that women and children in our society often behave in a passive manner does not necessarily support the view that they are inherently passive in nature. That the power which men have held over women is less easily demonstrated to be part of a natural order than that of the parent over the child has, of course, led to its being challenged in recent times. Nevertheless the beliefs derived from this power die hard.

The myth of male superiority is so ubiquitous and well-established that the phallus has become the symbol of life, value, and activity; the most positive feminine acts, such as childbirth and breast-feeding, being assessed in terms of their capacity to symbolise phallic failure or success. Although phallic idealisation may, to some extent, be a defensive compensation for envy of real feminine creativity—as some psychoanalysts, notably Melanie Klein, have suggested—valuation of the latter remains repressed and relatively ineffective as a factor in personality formation in societies in which the phallic myth prevails. The consequences of the myth, however, reflect not only on sexual development but on nonsexual infant rearing, and I shall first consider the latter.

Infantile Passivity

The infant is born into a human environment in which, according to his luck, one of two very different conceptions of him prevails. If his parents assume that he has a natural capacity for realistic perception and action, that he is a being whose views are to be treated with respect, they will watch him and listen to him, and try to respond accordingly to the messages he gives them, and will provide a medium in which he has sufficient room to express himself, to imagine, to create, to grow. They will—insofar as they are successful—protect him from everything that is irrelevant to and which interferes with the natural pace and manner of his growth. In short, they will respond to his advances as to a separate being, a real person, whose potential is as yet unknown but which they will endeavour to assist him in fulfilling. If however, the child finds himself in a world which has already made up its mind about him, which assumes him to be in a state of passivity waiting to be acted upon, his approaches will be met by responses that are geared, not to his individual nature, but to an alien and rigid system that meets his needs only at certain fortunate points. This occurrence may depend on fortuitous circumstances—he may be an unwanted child, be of the wrong sex, be conceived to replace a child who has died, or indeed be the recipient of all or any of the family's conscious and unconscious hopes and fears; but if he is born into a society which believes that infants are, or should be, passive, his chances of a receptive hearing are slight.

Active and Passive Development

The child whose native capacity for action is ignored or suppressed is like a blank sheet of paper waiting for the application of the print; his body will feel like an inert mass upon which patterns—pleasant or painful—are weaved by external forces, or a receptacle which needs to be filled or emptied from time to time. In these circumstances the skin, external orifices, and sensory mental processes will achieve undue importance and such remaining power of action that the child possesses will concentrate on incorporation and acquisition; resulting, psychologically, in the 'introjection' of the external world.

A confusion exists about the concept of introjection in that the term is used to describe not only the passive (pathological) mechanism described above but the normal and healthy process by means of which the child's psyche develops as a result of his relationship with his parents and other admired and important persons in his life. It is likely that the main reason for this confusion lies in the fact that in our society—and to an even greater extent in the society in which psychoanalysis first developed—the child is forced into a passive mould with the consequence that his psychic structure becomes overloaded with parental images.

Healthy psychic growth is the gradual unfolding of the basic, unique core of the child's experience and can only arise from an *active* and total functioning of his whole being in relationship with others. His belief in his perceptual experience rests on his trust of his own physiological functioning, even though this experience is made possible and coloured by the family and society into which he is born, and which he is bound in many ways to imitate. What is taken into the psyche from his experience with others is the memory of it, a memory which includes not only his perception of the other and of the other's structuring of the situation, but his own active participation and its effect. This memory enlarges his potential and increases his security, not because he thereafter carries with him an 'introject' like a magic charm but because in making an active and successful approach to another he has revealed the rich possibilities of interaction of which he and others are capable.

Whether this happy outcome of the interaction will occur depends, in the first place, on the attitude of the other person, who is usually his parent. If the parent sees and manipulates the relationship in such a way that the child is merely a passive recipient of his action, the experience gives the child no guarantee of future success in life except that bestowed by the arbitrary grace of the parent. The child can psychologically survive either in the presence of his parent, or, in his absence, by the memory that he has a parent capable of taking over his own functions, a circumstance readily depicted by the presence in his psyche of a powerful parent-image. An important element in this experience is that the relationship is a unique one; since the child is no more than the imprint of the parent's pattern, he is seduced into a position in which he is passively dependent on the other person's knowledge of this pattern and, moreover, the parent who operates in this omnipotent fashion conveys the impression of being uniquely different from anyone else whom the child may chance upon. In cases of excessive (psychotic) passivity one can often see that the parents have not only set themselves up as omnipotent but have sabotaged the child's attempts to find alternative relationships. As a consequence of such a state of affairs the child's real capacity to establish relationships with ordinary people atrophies or fails to develop. Although secondary—in time—to that of the parent, the child's defensive contribution to the eventual sterility is of comparable importance, consisting of his masochistic avoidance of hate and passive parasitic gain.

In a healthy parent-child set-up the parent provides a medium in which the child has sufficient room to focus his perceptions and express himself, a realistic reciprocation of the child's action, and a recognition that the parents' participation is not of exclusive importance. The consequence of this is that the child develops a realistic estimation of what he is like and can look to his parents as models to imitate, safe in the knowledge that they are providing a line of behaviour which may be shared by many people, including the child, a way of life that will prove its usefulness outside the family, rather than an exclusive and special performance (cf. Lomas[7]). (Stability, it is true, can result from the introjection of a myth of exclusive familial, racial, or sexual power—for instance, from 'blue blood' or 'white skin'—but such an illusion is increasingly difficult to maintain in the modern world. Diminishing comfort in pride of descent is perhaps one of the prices of increased knowledge.)

The Development of Sexual Identity

In spite of the importance of sexuality in human living there appears to be no reason to assume that the acquisition of sexual ability and identity is dependent upon circumstances any different from those that lead, or fail to lead, to the development of the rest of the personality (or, for that matter, that sexual factors are of unique significance). If the natural sexual urges are met by a realistic response and understanding, it seems likely that normal sexual development will take place. In a society that has become confused about the nature of its sexes, however, this cannot take place.

The phallic myth and its counterpart, the myth of female passivity and moral superiority, result from the rivalry between the sexes and constitute a kind of war or game in which the child is a pawn. The father sees his son as an extension of his own potency and power, someone of whom he is proud—provided he stays in his place—and whose advent he glorifies by childbirth rites in which the mother is, by and large, given a secondary or nonexistent part; the mother sees her son as a chance to obtain vicariously some of the male power she lacks, someone who must be wrenched from his father's grasp and brought under her influence.

In order to acquire real identity—including sexual potential—the boy must be capable of uninhibited perception of himself and others, a capacity which, in the circumstances described above, involves opposition to the fundamental tenets of his parents. If he accepts the sexual myth he not only denies his own perceptions but is himself drawn into a crippling struggle for power and prestige involving a fight with the other males of the family for possession of an elusive, idealised, and unsharable quality and a contemptuous attitude towards women with consequent fear of their real and imagined envy and revenge. If, on the other hand, he challenges the myth, he faces the anxiety and opposition of his parents and a recognition of the fallibility and confusion of those on whom he so much depends.

Several myths and fantasies are adopted as defence measures by children in attempts to solve their own individual problems, and such defence measures have received detailed attention by psychoanalysis—to a much greater extent, in fact, than the defences and mythologies of their parents—but to what extent these defences would occur or maintain their content in a society which had a more realistic view of sexuality is difficult to assess. A similar problem is presented by the question as to whether certain sexual and aggressive drives are innate or socially conditioned, notably incestuous desire. The intense oedipal rivalry to be observed in our society receives force from

   a. a spurious conflict propagated by the sexual myth;
   b. a healthy attempt to destroy the myth and break through to reality; and,
   c. seductive sexual manoeuvres by the parent designed, not merely to release sexual desire, but to prevent the child from seeking a loved object outside the family, thereby solidifying the myth of the 'Special Family.'

Incestuous seduction of this kind is in contrast to the healthy sexual feelings that can arise between parent and child and which include recognition of the necessity for renunciation, the occurrence of which has been so well described by Searles.[8]

This unrealistic presentation of life affects the girl at least as much as the boy and is not, of course, confined to the sexual realm. It rises from a view of existence in which people and things are valuable not because of their actual, perceptible, intrinsic qualities but according to a preconceived scale which meets with universal acceptance.

The Nature of Action

Action, according to psychoanalytical theory, is consequent upon drive or instinct, that is, it has its origin in the id, a specific part of the organism. It is likely that this conception is based on the Cartesian equation of self with reflective capacity, a notion which forces the conclusion that action derives from a somewhat alien part of the personality; but this conception has been seriously threatened in recent times (see, for instance, MacMurray[9]). Those writers who, like Fairbairn[10] and Rycroft[11] lay stress on the primary integration of the infant, would, therefore, not only appear to be suggesting a more manageable theoretical framework for a psychoanalytic theory of development, but would appear to be on firmer philosophic ground.

In this changed orientation the term 'action' is best used to describe the most adequate outcome of the total aims of the person which any given set of circumstances permits. It is the expression of what the person is—his identity—and the change which this person initiates in the world bears his unique mark, primarily meaningful within a personal context.

The Nature of Passivity

Inaction—the opposite of action—occurs when a person abandons a desired and realistic aim. His substitute behaviour takes on the quality of secondary activity, involves a sacrifice of identity and a degree of dissociation, and therefore approaches towards impersonal (vegetative, mechanistic) activity. But this does not apply, of course, if the original aim is abandoned in favour of another, more satisfactory, one. Complete inactivity probably does not occur in ordinary living but it may be reached in states which precede death, as may happen in extreme conditions of mental or physical illness or in the *Musselmanner* of the concentration camps. Elements of activity exist, firstly, to the extent that the original aim of expressing identity has not been entirely abandoned (although it may have been repressed), and secondly, insofar as areas of personality continue to operate autonomously in pursuit of secondary aims.

There are three different meanings to the word passive: (1) it is a synonym of 'inactive'; (2) 'quiescent'; and (3) 'submissive.' It would appear that in psychoanalytic literature the term has been used with the last of these three meanings in the forefront of the writer's mind. A passive person has been depicted not simply as one who does not act at all but one who acts in a certain manner, someone who, by such measures as submission to the other's authority or appeals to his pity and sense of guilt preys parasitically on his power, thereby gaining benefits and gratifications without direct effort on his own part. The essential feature of this manoeuvre is that the gains are acquired at the expense of autonomy and primary capacity.

The infant, unknowingly and of necessity, delegates many of the tasks of living to others until he has acquired the capacity to take them on himself. Paradoxically, one of the characteristics of growth—in both individual and society—is an increasing capacity to delegate tasks to others and to organise the physical environment so that it will perform tasks in such a way that freedom to develop and to live more richly is enhanced. The criterion of the fruitfulness, in both child and adult, of such behaviour is the degree to which immediate, direct action has been foregone without real loss of potential. It may be that one of the failings of our present society—as exemplified by the family studied in this chapter—is that too great a sacrifice of this kind is being made, that in seeking too good a reliance on things outside himself (money, opinion, status, physical safety, etc.) contemporary man has become passive and is teaching his child passive ways. He relies, and prides himself, not on his primary, spontaneous action and zest for life, but on his careful and watchful control of the environment so that his weakly self may be safe. The parents are, in this way, omnipotent; the ideal father earns money and the ideal mother protects her child from any possible disquieting or disturbing experience.

It would seem therefore that the essential feature of passivity—as the term is used both in ordinary language and in psychoanalytical writing—is parasitism. What is important is that it should be clearly distinguished from receptivity with which term it has been confused. Receptivity is, like parasitism, a type of dependence on another person, but it is characterised by a searching expectancy and capacity for gratitude. In almost every way it is quite the opposite kind of attitude from a parasitic one.

Active and Passive Identity

Those who conceive the primary integration of a being who is the agent of his own actions require an unambiguous term to denote the person about whom they are speaking, but there does not appear to be such a term readily available. Perhaps 'person' would be the best; the one most in use, 'self,' has a confused history in psychoanalytic theory and its rehabilitation has become difficult; a further alternative is 'identity.'

One disadvantage of the concept of identity is that, although Erikson, who introduced the term into psychoanalysis, stated that it originated in infancy, he focused his attention on adolescence with the result that the term has sociological overtones. More recently, Lichtenstein[12] has explored the infantile origins of identity, but in so doing he makes the—to my mind unnecessary—discrimination between an early 'identity theme' and a later 'identity.' Moreover, he fails to make the necessary distinction between active and passive identity. He writes:

> we must demonstrate how the human infant acquires an identity. I see the answer to this question in the 'imprinting' of an identity on the human child by the mother. The mother does not convey a sense of identity to the infant but an identity: the child is the organ, the instrument for the fulfillment of the mother's unconscious needs. Out of the infinite potentialities within the human infant, the specific stimulus combination emanating from the individual mother 'releases' one, and only one, concrete way of being this organ, this instrument. This 'released' identity will be irreversible, and thus it will compel the child to find ways and means to realise this specific identity which the mother has imprinted upon it.

This description, in fact, gives the impression of being an account of the kind of mother-infant relationship, typical of our society, which, I imagine, was experienced by my patient and which was an important factor in the formation of his passive character.

What is omitted in this conception—yet crucial to the theory of infantile development—is the distinction between active and passive identity, or, to put it in terms used (albeit with distinct connotations) by Winnicott and Laing, between the 'real' and the 'false' self system.

Conclusions

Stated briefly and dogmatically, the conclusions of the foregoing line of thought are as follows:

1. Passivity is not a specifically sexual phenomenon. It constitutes an abnegation of natural, authentic development and its substitution by a parasitic mode of existence in which reliance is placed on magic identification with an idealised entity.

2. Passivity is the fate of a child who is reared in a human environment (the family) which, instead of providing a suitable medium for growth, discourages action and rewards parasitism.

3. Although a particular family may act in this suppressive way for its own peculiar reasons, there are, in our society, general considerations liable to cause it to do so. Rigid dogma and myth prevent the family from perceiving the child as he really is; or, if it does so perceive him, it regards him as a potentially disturbing myth-destroyer who needs to be rendered innocuous.

4. The myth that is most relevant to this subject is that of the passivity (and, by implication, inferiority) of the woman and the child as opposed to the man. The consequence of this myth is that the woman and the child are moulded into a passive role while the man becomes engaged in a search for a spurious, idealised identity. The usual outcome of this perceptual distortion is not psychiatric illness but culturally syntonic character neurosis.

5. This myth has led to errors in psychoanalytic theory. These errors include faulty conception of activity, passivity, and identity, and of the distinction between real and false identity; the belief that identity develops primarily as a result of identifications (rather than through realistic interaction in a personal medium); an underestimation of the pathogenic effects of parental attitudes and a consequent overestimation of the importance of innate factors; and an unnecessarily large divergence between the theories of male and female development.

References

1. Winnincott, D.W. (1958), 'Metapsychological and Clinical Aspects of Regression within the Psychoanalytic Set-up,' *Collected Papers*, Tavistock, London.
2. Rycroft, C. (1951), 'A Contribution to the Study of the Dream Screen,' *Int. J. Psychoanal.* 32.
3. Fenichel, O. (1955), 'The Symbolic Equation: Girl=Phallus,' *Collected Papers*, 2d. series, Routledge, London.
4. Schachtel, E. (1959), *Metamorphosis*, Basic Books, New York.
5. Lomas, P. 'The Concept of Maternal Love,' see ch. 12.
6. Hermann, I. (1935), 'The Use of the Term "Active" in the Definition of Masculinity,' *Int. J. Psychoanal.* 16.
7. Lomas, P. (1962), 'The Origin of the Need to be Special,' *Brit. J. Med. Psychol.* 35.
8. Searles, H. (1959), 'Oedipal Love in the Countertransference,' *Int. J. Psychoanal.* 40.
9. Macmurray, J. (1957), *The Self as Agent*, Faber, London.

10. Fairbairn, R. (1952), *Psychoanalytic Studies of Personality*, Tavistock, London.
11. Rycroft, C. (1963), 'Beyond the Reality Principle,' *Int. J. Psychoanal.* 43.
12. Lichtenstein, H. (1961), 'Identity and Sexuality,' *J. Amer. Psychoanalytical Assoc.* 9.

4

Some Thoughts on Family Relationships in Contemporary Society

> *In the morning, to my relief, you are ugly. Monday's wan breakfast light bleaches you blotchily, drains the goodness from your thickness, makes the bathrobe a limp, stained tube flapping disconsolately, exposing sallow decolletage. The skin between your breasts a sad yellow. I feast with the coffee on your drabness. Every wrinkle and sickly tint a relief and a revenge. The children yammer. The toaster sticks. Seven years have worn this woman. The man, he arrows off to work, jousting for right-of-way, veering on the thin hard edge of the speed limit. Out of domestic muddle, softness, pallor, flaccidity: into the city....*
> —John Updike, 'Wife-wooing'

Lewis Mumford ends his book *The Condition of Man* with the words:

> In time, we shall create the institutions and the habits of life, the rituals, the laws, the arts, the morals that are essential to the development of the whole personality and the balanced community: the possibilities of progress will become real again once we lose our blind faith in the external improvements of the machine alone.

This chapter is a revised version of 'The Study of Family Relations in Contemporary Society' in *The Predicament of the Family*, edited by P. Lomas, Hogarth and the Institute of Psychoanalysis (1967).

> But the first step is a personal one: a change in direction of interest *towards* the person. Without that change, no great betterment will take place in the social order. Once that change begins, everything is possible.[1]

Mumford's plea is not, in our age, a lone one. Many writers—the most influential being Marx—have, in their various ways, stated their belief that the human being is, in both theory and practice, excluded from his rightful position. One might have expected that the recent spread of interest in psychology would place the person at the centre of affairs, but in this area of study the protagonist of the drama has been little in evidence and here, too, a defence of his rights has become necessary. Psychology strays from its authentic focal point in two ways: in the first the person is fragmented into a collection of drives, quotients, and body parts; in the second he is lost without trace in the group and becomes a unit or role.

To avoid these errors it is necessary to study a person directly and as a whole, and (since our concern is not with dead persons), in the active state of full participation in life. But when do people participate most naturally in life? In what circumstances can we see them as they really are? A distinction must be made between the actuality and potentiality of the person's existence. A man serving a life sentence is in his natural, normal state inasmuch as it is the one to which he is accustomed and has adapted, but is not a state likely to reveal much of his potential.

The psychoanalytic situation might seem at first sight to be as artificial as that of the routine psychological test (e.g., the presentation of the Rorschach card): the person is asked to lie on a couch, to give his associations, and the ordinary happenings that occur in social intercourse are avoided. The mitigating feature of this set-up, however, is the recognition by the analyst that in addition to such technical operations as, say, the interpretation of dreams, there exists a personal relationship between the two people, the experiencing and understanding of which is vitally important. Because the person is being studied in the context of a relationship, he is, to a large extent, seen in his natural habitat; his characteristic ways of dealing with people can be observed. Furthermore, insofar as inhibiting factors in his capacity for relating are successfully interpreted, his potentiality for experience with others will become manifest. Despite this, the analytic relationship remains one in which full development in certain directions is barred: the analyst is not a parent, spouse, or lover.

Another situation—perhaps an ideal one—which could be expected to yield accurate information about a person's real nature is that in which he is living with those most familiar to him: his family. But the degree to which his true self is revealed by a study of his family life will depend on the nature of his relationships in this sphere of life. A secure and happy family atmosphere will permit the emergence of the most open, passionate, and sensitive states of which he is capable; by contrast, what may be most in evidence are the defences that he has erected against what has hurt him most in his life. It would seem therefore, not unrealistic to hope that such a study could provide a rich source of information on both the positive and negative qualities of a person.

This line of thought provokes the question: 'Although the observation of the individual in the psychoanalytic situation has proved an immensely rewarding field of research, may not the study of the person within his family be an even better one?' In considering this question, however, it has to be noted that the two situations are not commensurate: the investigator in a therapeutic relationship with the family may be faced with technical problems more complex, and less known, than those of the analyst in his consulting room. On the other hand, certain techniques are more possible: he may even—a Malinowski among the Tobriand islanders—go and live with the family for a while, and get a firsthand experience of what life is like within it. Whatever the difficulties, there is clearly a relatively untapped source of wealth in this field.

Although Freud studied individuals in a setting away from their homes he managed to learn quite a lot about their families. He discovered that the impact of family life on the child was incomparably greater than had hitherto been suspected and he charted those patterns of conflict, most of which centred on family relationships, to be observed in the majority of his patients, and believed by him to have universal significance. His main themes (in this area of study) include the following:

1. The emotions aroused in the child by his natural relationships with parents and siblings, especially those deriving from physical contact, are the prime factors in moulding his personality.
2. The child experiences a passionate physical desire for his parents (especially the one of the opposite sex) even to the extent of desiring sexual intercourse, a wish that is counteracted by a phytogenetically deter-

mined incest bar. Ravaged by incestuous desire he directs a jealous hatred towards (in particular) the parent of the same sex as himself.
3. The natural authority of the family lies with the father, and he (and his sons) are inevitably envied by the females of the household.

Those who have continued to follow Freud's path of exploration have found for themselves that conflicts centred on these themes do really exist in the minds of their patients and are not confined to well-to-do Viennese at the turn of the century. This does not mean, however, that Freud was necessarily correct in his theories about the ultimate source of these conflicts. It is, in fact, unfortunate that the whole discipline of psychoanalysis is often judged on a particular detail of Freud's thinking, for instance, that the Oedipus complex is innate and not culture-bound. His assumption that the conflicts he unveiled are natural, inevitable and relatively independent of the actual family situation and prevailing philosophy of life was unwarranted and has encouraged psychoanalysts to neglect these latter factors.

Although psychoanalysis has been concerned primarily with the patient's fantasy system, clinical work published in recent years reveals an increasing recognition of his family as it is, and was, in reality; an attempt is now often made to create a picture of the parents as they really were and to use such knowledge in helping the patient to understand how he has come to behave in his characteristic way.

The retrospective study of family relationships which takes place in psychoanalysis is open to the criticism of being unreliable; such evidence, it is said, must be biased, is second hand, and the real events have been lost in the mists of time. To a degree, such a criticism is unanswerable, but it has to be remembered that all evidence is suspect and we have to collect our data where we find it and as best we can—even 'reliable, firsthand' data can often be a distortion of the subject's or observer's mind. The psychoanalyst, moreover, usually comes to know his patient fairly well, to allow for typical perceptual failures, and consequently to gain a reasonably accurate appreciation of the people in his life.

Psychiatry has always undervalued the capacities of the patient, has tended to regard his views as at worst, meaningless, or at best, the unbalanced and exaggerated preoccupations of an oversensitive soul—in any event, the views of an unreliable witness. And the patient undergoing psychoanalysis has not escaped this judgement. In part, no doubt, the fact that the psycho-analyst is preoccupied with the patient's distorted, as opposed to valid, perceptions leads him to take such a view, but one suspects that a question of status is involved: that the therapist is unconsciously betrayed into an assumption of superiority of judgement, and the patient's capacity for accurate perception is correspondingly marked down. If this prejudice were to be overcome, the evidence gained from patients about their families might be taken more seriously.

In the past decade or so there has been a new approach to the study of the family: the therapist or investigator conceives of the family as a single unit and observes all members together. A school of thought has grown around this method; centred in America it has its own style and technique. Although many, perhaps most, of those who operate in this way are psychoanalysts, they do not report their findings in psychoanalytic terms. Most of the families so far studied have contained a 'schizophrenic' member, and it is in relation to this enigmatic disorder that the approach has been most fruitful.

What is suggested by this work is that schizophrenia develops in a child who has been confused by his parents in their defensive attempts to maintain themselves. In such a family there is a gross failure of communication between members with the consequence that the child has little chance of developing a coherent and realistic picture of himself and his parents; his perceptual framework is built on shaky ground.*

The existence of this kind of family interaction is surely among the most important discoveries of psychiatry even though little is known about the exact development of such a malignant system, and the techniques which have helped to explore it are bound to become influential in our approach to the family. Already the way of thinking developed by these workers is being used to formulate family interaction in general. As Jackson has pointed out, the language used to describe intrapsychic states can deal only inadequately with the inter-

---

* Two early and important conceptions go by the name of 'double bind' and 'pseudomutuality.' In the former (Bateson et al.[3]) the child is stringently exposed to conflicting parental commands — one at the verbal, one at the non-verbal level. In the latter (Wynne et al.[4]) which receives further discussion in chapter 4, recognition of his individuality is replaced by blind preoccupation with a stereotyped role-relationship. A vivid account of several schizophrenic families characterized by communication failure has been given by two workers, Laing and Esterson,[5] who add their own individual theoretical orientation.

personal relationships of a family in action.² The school of thought discussed here has attempted to meet this problem, and perhaps Haley, one of its most lucid and original members, may best speak for himself. In the process of formulating intrafamilial exchanges, he cites, as illustration, this hypothetical example:

> The ideal child would misbehave in some way, for example, by leaning down and looking under the table. The father would speak to the child and tell him to straighten up. Mother would then speak to father and tell him he should not have chastised the child at that time or in that way. Father would say he was merely reprimanding the boy because it seemed necessary, and mother would look exasperated with him.

If someone were to try and improve the situation by persuading the child not to misbehave, the system would not alter. There would merely be a change of content.

> .... father is then likely to say to the child 'Why are you so quiet?' and mother will respond with 'He can be quiet if he wants, leave him alone' and father will say, 'I was only wondering' and mother will look exasperated. That is, a change in one individual can lead only to an adjustment, perhaps a relabelling of her behaviour, so that the system remains unchanged.

Haley's theoretical model for this kind of behaviour is a cybernetic one. He believes that

> People associating together during long periods of time will not put up with any and all kinds of behaviour from each other: they will set limits upon one another: insofar as family members set limits for one another, it is possible to describe their interactions in terms of the self-corrective processes in the total system. The family members respond in an error-activated way when any individual exceeds a certain limit. This process of mutually responsive behaviour defines the 'rules' of the family. In this sense the family is a system which contains a governing process. However, there is not just a single governor for the system; each member functions as a governor of the others and then the system is maintained.⁶

Using this kind of formula the ways in which family members manipulate each other, and the subtle modes of communication they utilize in so doing, can be studied with great effect. Haley's fictitious family, however, is a static one and is using mechanisms, which, in the individual, we would describe as defensive, obsessional, omnipotent, self-destructive, and so forth. There would appear to be a danger, which has its parallel in the field of individual psychology, that language found useful in the study of sick and sterile behaviour in families is asked to serve as a basis for the conception of healthy and creative states as well. Reading this kind of account one begins to feel that life is a complicated game and all that is necessary is to learn the correct rules and the best ways of handling people. What is omitted from this conception is the kind of atmosphere or medium which allows family members to contemplate each other in a nonmanipulative way and in which really spontaneous and creative relationships can develop.

[Note: Since writing the above, family therapy based on systems analysis has gone from strength to strength, and has become much more sophisticated in theory and technique. It is now a rich source of knowledge and ideas. The diversion from individual therapy remains striking even though many practitioners are trained in both disciplines. Whereas systems-therapy remains stubbornly impersonal—insofar as this can be managed—individual therapy remains focused on the personal, intimate relationship between practitioner and client. Perhaps this is inevitable, for a family is not an individual. But I am still inclined to the view that systems-analysis leaves a dimension untouched and that, if family therapy is to develop creatively, the question of intimacy between helper and helped must be confronted more that it is at present.]

How successful is the family? Is the present-day home a place wherein people are happy and fulfil their potential? Statistics give us an idea of the degree of overt failure—'problem families,' divorce, separation, neglect, mental or psychosomatic illness, criminality, delinquency, and so on. But are these manifestations merely the tip of the iceberg of distress? Psychoanalysis has shown that, because of the need to conceal it, failure exists on a wider scale than is commonly thought, often revealing itself, in negative and undramatic form, through a crippling restriction of endeavour and creativity. This criticism of the family is not made in any spirit of pessimism. It does not imply that these conditions are inevitable; that, for instance, the widespread ill-health and unhappiness in families is the consequence of genetic failings or of drives doomed to frustration; that, as Plato suggested, the family is intrinsically an evil and pathogenic organisation and the rearing of children best left to the state; or, that there is any substitute for parental love.

The evidence of psychoanalysis and related disciplines suggests that certain ways in which the family may fail to provide the child with the kind of psychological environmental he needs perpetuates an undesirable pattern:

1. The child is not given enough reliable, affectionate fondling to satisfy his sensuous needs.
2. His attempt to form an accurate picture of reality (including himself) is vitiated by the confusing way in which it is presented to him by others.
3. His capacity to express and receive emotional experience is dulled or crushed by discouraging responses from others;
4. No clear, if broad, path of development is marked out for him and no suitable leader exists on whom he can model himself.

The factors contributing to an unreceptive, rigid, defensive atmosphere stifling to the child are likely to be many and the task of unravelling them a formidable one. Perhaps the most one can hope to achieve is the unmasking of certain malignant patterns. But it is important to search in the most fruitful areas. Should we inspect the social organization in which families function or should we question our whole conception of the nature of family relationships?

One clue which may be of use in the search for conditions predisposing to family failure is the degree to which sick families—particularly those in which schizophrenia has developed—are isolated from society. In such families communication with outsiders is discouraged or prevented and a private and unsound culture incapable of rearing a citizen of the world flourishes. Could such a family manifest, in an exaggerated form, a condition of isolation that is endemic to our society and whose causes are traceable?

Historians and sociologists agree that in Western civilisation the family unit has become a comparatively small one, that the extended multigenerational family is now reduced to the nuclear two-generational one. Has this led to isolation? Further more, many families no longer live in tightly knit local communities where everyone knows everyone else. Although most families in our society are not socially isolated and maintain a complex network of social relationships with people and institutions, some cut down their external relationships to a degree that would be impossible in small-scale non-industrial societies.

In studying families as they exist in Britain, Bott discovered a correlation between families' internal and external relationships.[7] Although all families were individuated and lived in social networks rather than groups, the type of network concerned varied from the two extremes of 'close-knit' and 'loose-knit.' Loose-knit networks are those in which only a few of the people whom the family knows are in close relationship with one another. Such a loose-knit network exerts very little social pressure on the marital couple to conform to a set pattern of behaviour; on the contrary, it forces the family members to cooperate with each other and develop their own standards.

By contrast, in close-knit networks there is more agreement on codes of behaviour. When persons from such a network marry, they tend to maintain previous relationships, unshared by their spouse. There is little emphasis on joint husband-wife activity and ideology, and each maintains a rigid, segregated, sex-determined role.

It would seem therefore that in contemporary society the chances of a family becoming not only socially isolated but also (particularly those living in loose-knit networks) more individuated are greater than in traditional societies. It does not follow from this that isolation is the inevitable state of large numbers of families. But insofar as it does occur it may well lead to excessive interdependence of family members and to an idealization of their mutuality. In a short but extremely interesting article in the *Listener* (31 May 1962), Stephen Coates argues that the modern family is liable to neurosis on this account, in contrast with 'joint' families in which 'recognizing, from the whole of his childhood experience, the interdependence for each on each, the man may more consciously and rationally choose cooperation in place of competition; altruism in place of destruction.'

If, however, one brings to this question a consideration of the *quality* of the communication between family and external world the problem becomes a complex one, a social study of which is extraordinarily difficult. May not a family with benefit achieve a relative isolation from the communications of a society that are superficial, false or restrictive? And may not the release from rigid, segregated sex-roles lead to more creative unions within the family?

The modern family would appear to be in a state not dissimilar from the *identity crisis* of adolescence, as described by Erikson,[*] a state characterized by confused attempts to adapt to a new environment and set of values. The individual beset by such a crisis may either survive it to attain a new integration or may fall sick, the outcome depending not only on his own capacities but on the amount of understanding and toleration shown him by society. May the families of our time need a similar degree of support?

---

[*] In making this comparison I do not mean to equate family and individual or to support the theory, proposed by Westermark and others, that the modern family has evolved from that of 'primitive' societies.

The alienated family (I am using the 'schizophrenic' family as a model) avoids penetration from the outer world, wrapping itself in secrecy and mystification. Overtly endorsing the current mores, it often presents a highly respectable and normal front and may even regard its members as so above moral reproach that contact with others will be liable to corrupt them. Closer inspection, however, reveals an unhappy and bitter atmosphere, a gross failure of communication between members, an incapacity to love and grow and a deep, if concealed, sense of shame. It would seem likely that such a family is concealing a real failure, from whatever cause, presenting a public face of normality or even super-respectability. And, given the original failure, the attempts at concealment are not surprising, for in such matters our society is an intolerant one and is less concerned with the real than the apparent.

There is a peculiar pattern of family relationship which therapists report with notable frequency: that of the 'overpossessive' mother and the 'inadequate' father. The terms used vary—'dominating,' 'overprotective,' 'phallic,' 'schizophrenogenic,' for the mother; 'weak,' 'passive,' 'distant,' etc., for the father—but a constant picture of excessive maternal influence remains. It is one which has been held responsible for many kinds of disability in the child. Can this pattern help us to understand what is wrong with the family at the present time? Elucidation of the question meets up with the difficulty which dogs so much social research—that of norms and values. How 'protective' does a mother have to be before she can justly be called 'overprotective'?

The search for security permeates contemporary thought and action. We are all insured and inoculated, and those in public life who are responsible for the care of others must answer for any inefficiency. To some extent this attitude is a mark of increased respect for the individual, but often the precautionary measures are undertaken in an obsessive way and in a spirit of self-justification rather than genuine concern. The 'overprotective' mother is not simply concerned with her child but with *her own concern* for the child.*

She overemphasizes her function, presenting an idealized caricature of a mother, one who is ceaselessly and unselfishly devoted to her

---

* I do not wish to imply that such a mother is entirely lacking in love for her child; one factor in her narcissism may be an inability to tolerate the love feelings which she really has.

children. It is the behaviour of an insecure person living in a home where she anticipates criticism.

The father, faced by such a zealous and formidable partner, may withdraw from the scene of her operations and either succumb to a general state of ineffectiveness, transfer his interests elsewhere, or maintain the position of an important figure in the household, but one that is not directly concerned with the children. He may become totally absorbed, for instance, in the role of family breadwinner. This last case can easily give rise to conceptual confusion, for such a father may maintain his *status* by exaggerating the importance of his function as provider (and, perhaps, as authority in financial and other similar matters), and thereby appear a strong, forceful parent, fulfilling a traditional role in a normal manner. Nevertheless, it might still be thought that he has abdicated from a natural right to commune with his children, and the evidence of psychoanalysis suggests that the evil consequences of this alienation are legion.

At first sight this pattern seems a contemporary one: the emancipation of women has upset the traditional family regime: the mother exerts her new authority in too strident a way and the father has not yet found a way of adjusting to his dethronement. But perhaps, although there is some truth in this, the matter is not as simple as that. Have the traditional father and mother, each functioning within his and her designated sphere, ever been effective parents? Is the malignant syndrome under discussion merely one (somewhat disorganized) particular version of a family system which, even in its stable, traditional form, concealed a mutually destructive struggle between the parents for power, resulting in the idealization of their respective roles? Insofar as the parents are involved in a battle for status in which the child is the pawn, he will become emotionally involved in their conflict, unable to leave them and develop a life of his own. In this way, interpersonal strife leads the family to isolate itself from society not only to conceal its shortcomings but because it is so preoccupied with itself. To what extent does this family system, in which authentic living is replaced by a pursuit of power and prestige, arise as a consequence of a wrong conception of the nature of men, women, and children?

In the interest of law and order, society needs to erect leaders invested with the authority to issue certain kinds of commands. In other words, leadership roles must be respected in order that leaders may function adequately and maintain their position for a reasonable time.

In actual societies this necessary respect for leadership roles appears to get out of hand. Leaders command and demand respect, not merely in their technical capacity but as persons; they are deemed superior beings, and qualities incidental to their functions and shared by others are similarly idealized. The consequence of this trend is that societies become hierarchical; and status and symbols of status are valued at the expense of human beings.

Whether, or to what extent, idealization of leaders is necessary in order to maintain the structure of society is a debatable point. But it is a tendency which does not appear to have achieved very happy results, and has been the means by which large numbers of people have been tyrannized. And some of the myths associated with it, e.g., the superiority of white skin, are still alive and well. The situation is further complicated by the fact that in a society in which the overtly pronounced ideal is equality of status (as in our present democracy) a myth may develop that such equality has been reached long before this becomes a fact. But irrespective of origin, the consequences, in addition to that of possible tyranny, are (1) a denigration of the qualities of the led and (2) a preoccupation with classification; people are not perceived as individuals but conceived as examples of classes. To what extent may these observations apply to the internal structure of the family? Are there divisions of a similar nature, to which we have become so accustomed that we regard them as natural and inevitable.

That parents, owing to their greater power, knowledge and technical ability, must be the family leaders is not in doubt. The question is whether, in their capacity as parents, they idealize themselves at the expense of the child. If this does occur, it may manifest itself by:

1. An open assertion of superiority, prior right, and unquestionable power and wisdom; or
2. a preoccupation with the importance of the child which conceals the fact that he is regarded as an extension of the parent and that his real nature and aims are being overlooked.

In many societies, the first of these manifestations applies—at least, as far as we can judge, using our own criteria. What is the case in our own society, in which children have been officially emancipated? May the second pattern be widespread, or, possibly, may the first exist to a greater extent than is commonly supposed, being disguised by a bland assertion that parents no longer dominate their children?

A confusion exists because authority is equated with arbitrary status. Insofar as the status of the parent rests on something over and above his real qualities a decrease in status is not necessarily accompanied by a decrease in authority; one might, in fact, surmise that a child's real respect for his parent will increase if the latter is open and unpretentious in his behaviour. The widespread belief that this kind of parental behaviour is harmful—that 'permissiveness' and encouragement of free expression lead to juvenile delinquency and the like—is perhaps due, firstly, to its being confused with the leniency that comes from weakness, and secondly, the assumption that such an attitude will inevitably be exploited by the child—an assumption, similar to that held by those of 'superior' status about their 'inferiors', which has doubtful validity. If a parent, unobstructed by individual or cultural bias, perceives the child realistically, he will be able to assess his capacity to take personal responsibility, that is, he will accurately understand both the childlike and adultlike qualities that are present and respond accordingly. The child, because he is thereby enabled to develop a healthy sense of identity, may not need to exploit destructively, and, in any case, will be confident that attempts to do so would meet with little success. On the other hand, children who exploit their parents, who become 'spoiled,' do so because their potentialities and limitations are not truly seen; both too little and too much is asked of them, and so they begin to strive for illusory rights and compensations for real deprivations. The parents may add to the confusion in their attempts to make up for their failure by further leniency and the provision of secondary pleasures, maintaining a self-idealization based on their tolerance and generosity. Thus what appears superficially to be an abdication of status on the part of the parent is in fact a failure to recognise the real nature of the child, and a battle for status takes place in which little self-expression is possible for either party. The creative and self-disciplinary response of which a child may be capable if he is respected as a person who is different from but equal in status to an adult is perhaps something that we do not often have the chance to witness.

In suggesting that parental self-idealization is an important source of trouble to families in our society I do not mean to imply a belief that parents need *never* present themselves in an idealized form to their children. Clearly a child should be preserved from unnecessary worry and confusion, especially when he is very young, and occasions arise when parents have to conceal their doubts from him (to the extent that this can be done without adding further confusion). But in some cases the deception will be conscious, minimal, and in tune with the child's requirement. And in infancy, when this kind of requirement is at its height, only the mother who is free from thoughts of her own role and status can be sufficiently spontaneous to provide it. By contrast, compulsive and rigid self-idealization is incompatible with the child's need for self-expression and exists for the wrong reasons. These include not only a desire on the part of the parents to preserve their status within the home in the face of the child's developing challenge but also:

1. Sadistic compensation for the deprivations and humiliations which they themselves have suffered in their lives;
2. Obsessional need to control all relationships and to prevent the emergence of a disturbing creative drive in the child;
3. The quest for respectability: parents who are insecure in their role require reassurance from the public that their house is in order.

When we come to consider the relative status of male and female within the family the problem, however confused, is clearer in one respect than the corresponding dichotomy of parent and child, for we are dealing with people of comparable ability.

That the male is superior to the female has been the overt assumption of most societies, irrespective of social structure.* Western civilization has seen a gradual advance in the status of women, but, although our legal system is an improvement over that of the code of Hammurabi, it still shows a masculine bias. Moreover, much casual and unconscious thinking in everyday life derives from an automatic acceptance of inequality between the sexes, and the suffering consequent upon this view is revealed by patients during psychoanalysis. Psychoanalysts themselves have not presented a clear theory of the origin of this belief and of the envy of women (which undoubtedly exists, if not to a comparable extent). But it is difficult not to give significance to so glaringly obvious a factor as the social climate in which children learn their values.

The question of woman's status is linked with that of the family as

---

* 'Favourable as the position of woman under mother-right appears on the surface,' wrote Hobhouse, 'the truth is that it is no bar whatsoever to complete subjection.'[10]

a whole since, rightly or wrongly, the two are equated in the public mind: 'a woman's place is in the home.' In compensatory defence the woman may deny the importance of family life and idealize typically masculine (professional and public) roles; or she may assert the supreme importance of motherhood and family life, with consequences discussed in the previous section: a reversal of roles may give prominence to a matriarchal tyrant.

In contemporary 'middle-class' as opposed to 'working-class' society in Britain the father has now become less of an authoritarian but more of a participant in home life—a change linked with the tendency towards loose-knit networks, noted above. And one would therefore suppose that there is a concomitant increase in psychological well-being in such a household. But whether this happy outcome has really taken place is debatable. Apart from the fact that such things are very difficult to measure there are reasons why a desirable result may not simply follow this changed pattern of relationship. First, the change may be more apparent than real, involving conscious but not unconscious experience; secondly transitional problems (e.g., the emergence of an unsatisfactory paternal norm of behaviour of the 'mother's help' variety) may dominate the scene; and thirdly, middle-class life often has additional characteristics (e.g., intellectual defences against spontaneity or the idealization of 'success') which may work against an improved emotional climate within the family. [Note: In spite of the fact that, since the above was written, far more mothers have careers and fathers (the 'new men') play a greater part in child-rearing, the mutual striving for power and status within the family has not visibly diminished. Indeed, the change may well have added a complexity which provides husbands and wives (and their lawyers) with more sophisticated armoury. The phenomenon is rather similar to the arguments, observed by the harassed marital therapist, between combatants whose knowledge of psychodynamics has merely sharpened their weapons.]

In the midst of this maze of possibilities one fact remains with a fair degree of certainty. A general improvement in psychological health can only be expected if and when children grow up in families in which they are treated with respect and sincerity as real and unique persons—in short, if they are loved. And this can only take place if society gives the family a chance to function in this way. I would suggest that, among the many reasons why this happens to only a limited extent at present, the following one is important: the work of the parent is not given similar status to other kinds of work requiring comparable time and skill since (a) it is considered to be the typical and traditional work of *women* and (b) it is existential, in the sense that it cannot be easily measured and marked and presented to the world in the shape of an unambiguous achievement. If this line of thought is correct then perhaps one should ask, not 'Has the family become alienated from society?' but 'Has society become alienated from the family?'

It is, in fact, appallingly difficult to communicate usefully about therapy because (a) there is no generally acceptable definition of health (and therefore of cure) and (b) those anxious to bring about a beneficial change in people's lives are, through human frailty, liable to overvalue their methods and results. Moreover, therapy can be adequately demonstrated only in cases where an accurate assessment has been made. By what means should a particular family be approached therapeutically? A possible road is via single members of the family. In this case the aim can be to influence one member in the hope that he, in turn, by means of fresh insights, better morale, or increased maturity, may help the family as a whole towards an improvement of some kind. But which member should be first approached: the apparently sick one, the most powerful, the healthiest? Can we expect better results if two therapists who are engaged in working individually with two different family members confer together and form a joint plan of campaign? Or should they refrain from influencing each other, as many psychoanalysts believe? Is it more fruitful to treat the family collectively? There are many other pressing questions that could be added, the answers to which remain unknown to us.

Psychoanalysis and related methods of therapy of similar complexity are sometimes condemned because their beneficiaries can only be few and must be fairly well-off financially. And it seems likely that an intense form of family therapy will be open to the same kind of criticism, a criticism which, at the present time, is a just one. But the importance of psychoanalysis rests not only on its therapeutic efficacy but its capacity as an instrument of research and as a stimulus of thought in many areas of life, and in particular, that of the family.

I will end with a few lines from Thomas Blackburn's poem for a Child:

And have I put upon your shoulders then,
What in myself I have refused to bear,
My own and the confusion of dead men,
You of all these, my daughter, made my heir,
The furies and the griefs of which I stayed
Quite unaware?

Postscript 1996

Any degree of optimism that found its way into this essay written thirty years ago, was, alas, unfounded. The family has never been more under threat than now. A greater awareness of the child's need for understanding and self-expression, so central a precept of that time, has not led to a poised adolescent, a happy, united family, or a flourishing society. Those who, like myself, had such hopes, however modest, were naive. It seems as though when one good emerges in a society (for instance, an increased psychological space for the child to develop into an autonomous being) other forces react in a way that brings fresh difficulties. We are, as yet, and possibly always will be, too ignorant of the whole to know how best to improve our way of living. I am reminded of the disturbance to the family system of a thoughtless but well-meaning therapeutic attempt to help one of its members in isolation—or, on a grander scale, of the effect on the total world environment of any single effort to change one aspect of nature. If one takes a look at the literature on the family of the past three decades it is difficult to find any consensus of what, in the main, prevents the family from being the secure base from which children could emerge with the confidence and balance to take their place in society. And it is equally difficult to grasp, among the babble of voices and opinions of the politicians and the sociologists, why society is in such bad shape to embrace these children. If one were to attempt to extract any agreed view, it would, I think, be that society has become too atomistic and that our values have shifted, with the help of the free market and advanced technology, from a sense of community to a focus on individual desires. Any attempt on my part, with no claim to any expertise beyond what occurs in my consulting room, is surely destined to the unhappy fate of so many expectations and predictions about the family. But we often attempt the impossible, and perhaps this is inevitable. I will, however, limit myself to one impression, for which I claim no originality.

The rivalries which Freud outlined appear to be an inevitable factor of our innate constitution and the circumstances of family life. And he is also undoubtedly right that an acceptance of the inevitability of these rivalries and of the many other unwelcome exigencies of living is crucial in our achieving stability and well-being. This conception stands as a solid base for any thoughts about the family and society. How best to help a child to handle those elements that resist his or her efforts to change them is the question with which we are faced. The psychotherapeutic revolution of this century has lead us to encourage the child to explore the limits of the possible and to make those limits as extensive as can be managed, thus fostering his creativity, autonomy, and exuberance of living. In recent years, however, a backlash has occurred and disciplined formality has returned to our schools, a move considered justified by the apparent failure of 'progressive' education and child-rearing.

Throughout this time, and including the present, the child has been subjected to mixed messages. The Protestant Ethic has never left us. We may adopt and embrace new ways of thinking, but these take time to affect our unconscious; archetypes are not transient. The consequence is that parents have themselves been confused and have therefore confused the child; there have often been wide discrepancies of ideology between the parents and the school, and between the generations. To place the ills of the family on this issue would be a gross simplification. What I aim to suggest, however, is that a coherent milieu for a child to grow with greater freedom of expression and communication than appears to have occurred in past centuries has never been achieved by contemporary society and therefore the ideas that have been expressed on this matter by psychotherapists and leaders in educational thought—including Dewey, Montessori, and Froebel—have not been shown wanting.

References

1. Mumford, L. (1963), *The Condition of Man*, Mercury Books, London.
2. Jackson, D. (1963), 'Comment,' *Family Process*, 2.
3. Bateson, G. et al. (1956), 'Towards a Theory of Schizophrenia,' *Behavioral Science* 1, 4.
4. Wynne, L.C. et al. (1958), 'Pseudo-Mutuality in the Family Relations of Schizophrenics,' *Psychiatry* 21, p. 205.

5. Laing, R.D. and A. Esterson (1964), *Sanity, Madness and the Family*, Tavistock, London.
6. Haley, J. (1963), *Strategies of Psychotherapy*, Grane & Stratton, New York and London.
7. Bott, E. (1957), *Family and Social Network*, Tavistock, London.
8. Zimmerman, C.C. (1947), *Family and Civilisation*, Harper, New York.
9. Erikson, E. (1959), 'Identity and the Life Cycle,' *Psychological Issues*, vol. 1, part 1, International Universities Press, New York.
10. Hobhouse, L.T. (1906), *Morals in Evolution*, Chapman & Hall, London.

5

Family Interaction and the Sick Role

In this chapter I shall discuss the ways in which the concept of illness, whether overtly physical or mental, can be utilised by the family in its attempt to solve the problems of cooperative living.

The Dynamics of Power within the Family

In an ideal family, just as in an ideal world, the participants would engage each other cooperatively in a venture that would lead to mutual benefit and growth. The families of our culture fall short of this ideal to a varying degree; cooperation is replaced by exploitation and a battle for power ensues. In the earlier days of history physical strength is likely to have been the dominating factor in this struggle but, in increasing degree, more sophisticated means of attack and defence are used. The weaker members—weaker in regard to physical strength, age, social status, and so forth—use various manipulative techniques to gain ascendancy. One of these techniques is the application of a moral code designed to benefit the weak, that is, themselves. According to such a code, weakness could be invested with high moral value, or alternatively identified as a state necessitating special consideration. This latter assertion clearly has a realistic biological basis, for a society that allowed indiscriminate exploitation of its weaker members, e.g., its children, would fare badly. However, the element of reality

---

Published in *The Role of Psychosomatic Disorder in Family Life*, edited by Wisdom and Woolf, Pergamon (1965)

can be exaggerated for the purpose of giving the weaker partner supreme power.

In our culture there is a defined role, that of being ill, wherein these considerations apply with particular force.* If any family member cannot by ordinary means gain or maintain the position of power that he wishes for or feels to be his right, the adoption of the sick role is a possible alternative method of attaining his desired goal. All he has to do is to convince the family that he has some unavoidable incapacity and, having attained this strategic position, to launch a counterattack on those in power. Such a move is similar to the deliberate sacrifice of a piece in chess and is, of course, no guarantee of success.

The sick person may add weight to the advantage accrued from this code by attempting to demonstrate that other people are, in fact, causally responsible for his unhappy state; that by cruelty or neglect or excessive demands they have reduced him to this condition. Since such assertions may not survive logical scrutiny they are usually conveyed by hints rather than overt statements, and if this manoeuvre is successful a family or cultural myth will develop. An example of this is the widespread and deep-seated belief that the woman's menstrual and child-bearing functions naturally and inevitably incur a multitude of physical and mental disabilities. This myth enables the woman to induce a belief in the man that his 'selfish' desire for sexual satisfaction is the cause of her ailments and to exploit his consequent sense of guilt in order to master him. She can only maintain this myth, however, at the expense of a denial of her sexual and maternal wishes.

The existence of a sick role has its uses not only to the potential occupier of this role, but to other members of the family who might wish to place him there. The social mobility of a daughter can, for instance, be greatly restricted if her mother, fearing her developing sexuality and possible defection, decides that she is delicate or nervous and needs a mother's care. This gambit can be even more effective if, by use of the concept of insanity, the perceptions of the 'troublesome' member of the family are deemed invalid, an example of which would be the questioning of the sanity of an ageing relative who decides to revise his will in a way unacceptable to family members.

---

* The nature of the sick role, especially insofar as it concerns the doctor-patient relationship has been discussed by Balint[1] and Talcott Parsons.[2]

An attempt may be made not only to *label* a family member insane, but, as Searles[3] has shown, to *drive* him insane.

The only difference, insofar as the psychodynamics of the family is concerned, between psychosis and other types of illness is one of degree. In other illnesses a measure of responsibility in family matters is maintained, sometimes even perversely enhanced; a role is still occupied within the family system. In psychosis the role is vacated and identity lost. Insofar as a psychotic can be thought of as still being in the game, his move is to relinquish his place as a last desperate plea that drastic action be taken to render his position tenable. In relation, therefore, to the concept of illness, two opposite manoeuvres are possible in the fight for ascendency: to be sick or to prove (or make) the other sick. Which manoeuvre will be adopted will depend on availability and utility of role.

Sadomasochism and Sickness

A factor common to the one who seeks a sick role and the one who needs to relate to a sick person is sadomasochism. The sick person gains masochistic pleasure from the contemplation of his suffering and sadistic satisfaction from his seductive control of others. The compulsive sick-attendant needs to believe that he has renounced happiness in favour of unselfish and sacrificial care of others yet basks in the power of his authority over the patient. This type of relationship, particularly as it involves patient and nurse or patient and therapist in hospital practice has been described by Main.[4]

A particular gambit, which both sick and attendant may use, is to seek the prestige that accompanies strength *and* weakness by possessing both qualities at once. The sick person shows strength by his fortitude in the face of suffering and the helper, by his ability to carry on in spite of not being really up to it, suggests that *he* is really the weak one. These moves are carried on by nonverbal communications, such as brave smiles and sighs of long-suffering and fatigue.

The Need to be Well

The compulsive need to be the (apparently) strong one vis-à-vis an invalid may arise, as has been suggested above, from an endeavour to gain ascendency in a battle for power and to find an outlet for sadistic impulses. The role of healer is, in addition, a useful means of dealing indirectly with a disturbing urge to be ill. Not only can reassurance be gained from the contrast with the sick one, but vicarious gratification occurs due to identification with him.

A description of a mother who compulsively needed to be the strong one is given by Jackson.[5] Describing the second interview with a thirty-year-old catatonic schizophrenic and her mother he writes: During the interview, the mother said that her husband was nervous and had periods when he was unable to go to work and when she took care of him. She also described how the patient's younger brother had had a similar spell just before leaving for Korea during the conflict there. The therapist asked the mother, since her husband as well as her son and daughter had had breakdowns, was she ever able to allow herself to let down or did she always have to be the strong one? The mother looked very confused, blushed, and finally stated: 'It's all over and there's no sense in going into it'; and 'It was just silly. It is past history.' Despite the therapist's telling her that with this attitude she could not possibly understand her daughter; furthermore that it was unfair to treat herself in this way, she still denied that her own 'breakdown' was of any importance and would not go into the matter. The therapist turned quickly to the daughter and asked her what her understanding of this was, and she replied promptly, though in a whisper, that her mother could understand other people when they had troubles but seemed unable to admit that she had any of her own. The mother then launched into a long apology for having left her daughter so much when she was an infant, and became tearful and admitted the extent of her difficulties with her husband in the early days of their marriage. The patient listened interestedly and upon questioning remarked that she had not been told of this before. She nodded, however, when the therapist stated that she must have had some inkling of it.' Jackson goes on to describe how, following the revelations in this session, the daughter not only showed considerable clinical improvement but began to manifest strength in relation to her mother who in turn became helpless and dependent.

The techniques whereby a person may be induced or seduced into disability are numerous and include the following:

1. To punish efficiency. Except in unusual circumstances (as, for instance, in certain situations in modern industry) this is not done overtly. A

child, however, may discover that the growth which diminishes his need for parental supervision brings their ill-favour.
2. To undermine the person's necessary confidence in his ability and health by repeated assertions of his inadequacy, by a failure of consensual validation, or by confusing him as to his intentions, capacities, effectiveness, and identity.
3. To take over functions of the person that are natural and appropriate to his status and capacity, thereby inducing laziness, atrophy of function, and an ever increasing and more paralysing indebtedness.
4. To render disability more socially acceptable by exaggerating and encouraging its capacity to amuse and endear. (This capacity is based on its incongruity, its potentiality as a releaser of sadistic tension in the other, and the reassurance gained from the repetition of a familiar pattern).

The Use of the Sick Role in the Preservation of Meaning and Respectability

The sick role is a convenient measure for maintaining the balance of power within the family and its value as a defence lies, in particular, in its avoidance of the naked truth of the situation. A family, the stability of which depends on the upholding of a myth of mutual love and concern, could not risk the unmasking of this myth by open conflict and the revelation of hate. The confusion which would result from sudden disillusionment would be terrifying to all members and must be avoided at any cost. The sick role offers a way out of this dilemma.

In sickness, an appearance of meaning and purpose is preserved; the doctor can be called, medicaments given, certificates written, and a respectable and guilt-saving cause of the disturbance is found. The form that the illness will take, and the extent to which it will be physical or mental will be influenced by the prevailing conception in the culture as to what constitutes a respectable illness. In our society mental illness is becoming increasingly acceptable, which perhaps accounts for the diminishing prevalence of conversion hysteria.

Sadistic exploitation can be veiled by unselfish caring for others, and unpredictable and frightening revelations can be rationalised as occurring only because of this new concept brought into the family dynamics: 'Sickness.' 'He only acts this way' it is said, 'because he is not well: he is not himself.' This rationalisation is most striking when the illness is psychosis, and it can be poignant to see parents who prefer to accept a diagnosis of insanity in their adolescent child rather than recognise the genuine hate and distress revealed by the child's utterances.

Not only the remaining family members but the patient can find relief in the sick role which preserves both himself and those he loves (however ambivalently) from the sharp edge of painful reality.

The Primary and Secondary Gain of Illness

Freud's view that the advantages incumbent upon falling ill are of only secondary etiological importance has been challenged by Szasz[6] in *The Myth of Mental Illness* in which he conceptualises hysteria as primarily a nondiscursive language brought into operation in situations in which ordinary language fails in its aims. He writes: 'Traditionally, the socially communicative aspects of neurosis were subordinated to the intrapsychic (intrapersonal) and unconscious aspects of it. Perhaps in an effort to give a kind of conceptual superiority to the latter, its achievements—for example, the satisfaction of sexual or pregenital impulses by means of a symptom—were called *primary gain*. This was contrasted with the *secondary* use (hence the name) to which the symptoms might have been put . . . .This distinction seems to me unnecessarily sharp. It fails to do justice to the exquisite intermingling of intrapersonal, interpersonal, and social levels of communication that characterise most human situations. Approaching our problems more operationally . . . the distinction between primary and secondary gain becomes increasingly unimportant.'

It would seem, however, that while accepting Szasz's criticism of the traditional differentiation between primary and secondary gain it may still be useful to maintain a distinction of a somewhat different kind. Primary gain could refer to the immediate advantage which adoption of the sick role gives to a person who finds himself in an intolerable situation, while secondary gain could be applied to the gradual and progressive adaptation to and exploitation of this role that comes with time and practice.

The Assumption of the Sick Role as a Temporary Therapeutic Measure

Hitherto in this chapter the adoption of the sick role has been considered as a form of family adaptation leading to a sterile and destructive sequence of events. However, sickness, in an individual, usually carries a potential for growth and the manifest symptoms contain, in distorted form, elements of the real nature of the person which have previously remained in repression. In certain types of illness, for instance, the *identity crisis* of adolescence described by Erikson,[7] during which abnormal and often alarming physical and mental phenomena occur, this has particular application. Winnicott[8] describes a temporary disintegration of personality, called by him a 'regression to the true self,' occurring in a therapeutic setting, which can lead, if managed correctly, to a further growth of personality.

With the help of these ideas it becomes possible to conceive the sick role as a temporary asylum, necessary in times of crisis and growth, by means of which ordinary commitments are avoided and the energy saved can be utilised for purposes of reorganisation. In fortunate cases the family may intuitively recognise and respond to this need, an event that is most likely to occur at adolescence or during pregnancy and the puerperium. It is doubtful if such individual organisation in a creative way could be allowed to occur without a corresponding growth in other family members. In some cases the family may attempt to precipitate a member into a breakdown not out of malicious intent, but to enable him to make use of the sick role in a productive way. In turn, the family unit itself may also be considered at times to adopt a sick role in relation to society, either destructively or as a temporary relief measure.

Conclusion

Insofar as the adoption of a sick role within a family is determined rather than accidental, it is done so because it offers a possible way of maintaining equilibrium in the face of impending disintegration. To the extent that preservation of a binding, rigid, and idealistic system is sought at the expense of individual autonomy, it is a defensive and destructive manoeuvre. In certain cases—and perhaps to some extent in many cases—it offers a temporary resting place and carries with it a potential for growth.

References

1. Balint, M. (1957), *The Doctor, his Patient and the Illness*, Pitmans, London.
2. Parsons, T. (1952), *The Social System*, Tavistock, London.

3. Searles, H.F. (1959), 'The Effort to Drive the Other Person Crazy—An Element in the Aetiology and Pathology of Schizophrenia.' *Brit. J. Med. Psychol.* 32, 1.
4. Main, T.F. (1957), 'The Ailment.' *Brit. J. Med. Psychol.* 30, p. 129.
5. Jackson, D.D. (1961), 'The Monad, the Dyad, and the Family Therapy of Schizophrenics,' in *Psychotherapy of the Psychoses*, edited by Arthur Burbon, Basic Books, New York.
6. Szasz, T.S. (1961), *The Myth of Mental Illness,* Hoeber-Harper, New York.
7. Erikson, E.H. (1956), 'The Problem of Ego Identity,' *J. Amer. Psychoanalytical Assoc.* 14, p. 56.
8. Winnicott, D.W. (1954), 'Metapsychological and Clinical Aspects of Regression within the Psychoanalytic Set-up,' in *Collected Papers* (1958), Tavistock, London.

6

Childbirth, the Family, and Breakdown

To have a baby is an event in a woman's life the psychological impact of which can hardly be exaggerated and which is accompanied by an important change in attitude to herself and to her family. At one particular point, the time of the birth itself, the changes of attitude required of her are sudden and dramatic, and can be briefly summarized as follows:

1. There are sudden, gross changes in the body image;
2. Fantasies of the baby are replaced by realities; whatever the conscious and unconscious expectations of him, he is now seen to be what he is and no more;
3. There is immediate need to make physical and emotional contact with a baby whose primitive demands remind the mother of her own repressed ones;
4. There is responsibility towards the baby. Up to the time of birth this responsibility was taken by the mother's body; now she herself has to soothe and nourish a being whose existence is precarious and whose needs are sudden and urgent.
5. Childbirth involves a change of status. In some cultures the first childbirth involves the mother in a change of name. Such a change may, like a Finals examination, be unconsciously regarded as the achievement of

---

This is a revised version of 'The significance of postpartum breakdown,' a chapter in *The Predicament of the Family*, edited by P. Lomas, Hogarth and the Institute of Psychoanalysis, London, 1967.

adulthood, with all the conflict which this may bring. She needs to be able to tolerate success.
6. The mother's relationship to her husband is altered. She has drastically to divide her loyalties and to rely on his cooperation and support in this;
7. She has to be able to allow herself to trust and depend on others, since she is now incapacitated, not only by body changes but by the chains of her baby's needs;
8. Childbirth often involves a sudden change in the environment, geographical and emotional, e.g., removal to hospital.

Although many of these events are more dramatic at the time of a first parturition, they also occur in successive ones.

With these hazards in mind, one can attempt a forecast of the kind of personality defect that would make a woman susceptible to a puerperal breakdown. She would be a woman who had failed to reach emotional maturity, whose conflicts prevented her from admitting to herself and others that she had reached adult, parental status and from acting with the responsibility required of that status; she would lack close touch with reality; incline towards idealistic expectations of childbirth, be unaware of her deeper emotional layers, that is, have repressed experience relating to the intense anxiety and danger involved in infantile crying or to the sensuous bodily feeling that accompanies, for instance, breast-feeding. Her degree of flexibility would be insufficient to enable her to adjust to the major and minor hazards that so often complicate even a 'normal' confinement. It is to be expected that a scrutiny of mothers suffering from puerperal breakdown would reveal the presence of these personality deficiencies, irrespective of the differences of approach and interpretation of the investigators.

In a study of puerperal breakdown at The Cassel Hospital many of these expected features were manifest. This series of mothers, who were treated by psychoanalytical-orientated therapy, excluded unmanageable psychosis owing to the nature of the setting, but contained a cross-section of psychiatric diagnoses, depression being the most frequently encountered.

The mother's personalities prior to breakdown, as seen in retrospect, revealed strong tendencies towards rigidity and masochism. Their relationship with their own parents was an unhappy one and they had taken little joy in life, repressing their spontaneity and femininity: they were sexually immature and—to a varying degree—frigid. Prior to the breakdown, much of their failure in personality development had been concealed from themselves, but now had become more difficult to ignore. This study grew out of a therapeutic endeavour and was not a controlled experiment. But although no controlled comparison was made with healthy puerperal mothers the lack of those characteristics necessary for successful mothering was clear and could be seen to contribute to the breakdown.

Psychoanalysts have not, on the whole, paid very much attention to this subject. Winnicott and Helene Deutsch have both studied maternity intensively, and much that they have written is relevant to a discussion of puerperal breakdown, but they have not focused on the illness itself. In a recent paper Douglas[1] gave a clinical presentation of a woman with postpartum depression, many of whose problems stemmed from an 'excessive compliance with the mother'—a sign of emotional immaturity and failure of identity development. For many years the only psychoanalytic study of postpartum breakdown was that by Zilboorg, and it is to his work that reference is usually made in psychiatric literature. His most frequently quoted findings, namely that frigidity is a significant precursor of the illness, found confirmation in our study and it was therefore surprising to discover that in several current psychiatric textbooks, and in a book devoted to the study of postpartum breakdown, Zilboorg's work is regarded as having been completely refuted. Hamilton writes:

> Throughout the recent psychiatric literature there is a recurrent theme: that sexual abnormality is a precursor and perhaps an important cause of postpartum psychiatric illness. This theme is expressed more succinctly and bluntly by Zilboorg, to the effect that the premorbid personality of puerperal mental patients is characterised by frigidity and by latent homosexuality. Zilboorg's opinion was based on analytic studies of a very small number of patients with well-developed schizophrenic syndromes.
>
> A different opinion has been expressed by other investigators who have approached the problem with statistical methods. When large numbers of postpartum cases were compared with other cases unrelated to child-birth, Anderson and others were unable to find an increased incidence of predisposing sexual difficulties among the puerperal cases.[2]

And, in *Clinical Psychiatry*, Mayer-Gross, Slater, and Roth write:

> Zilboorg has stressed the part played by psychological conflicts and the attitude towards husband and child in the aetiology of these psychoses (i.e., puerperal). But Anderson, using a series of controls, has rebutted many of his claims. That prenatal hygiene, desirable as it is, should be able to prevent psychosis after childbirth is not to be expected.[3]

How have such differences of opinion arisen? There would seem to be two main reasons: a confusion about the phenomenology and terminology of 'frigidity,' and a misunderstanding of the way in which psychological factors have significance in the causation of mental illness. Before considering these problems it is necessary to look at Zilboorg's findings in a little more detail.

Zilboorg made a pioneering study of the psychodynamics of puerperal breakdown and reported his findings in four papers.[4] He was a psychoanalyst and he focused his attention on those matters that were of chief interest to psychoanalysts at the time when he was writing, namely, sexual drive and unconscious fantasies on physical desire, particularly in so far as these centred on the 'Oedipus complex.' Although much of his papers was descriptive, he couched his discussions and conclusions strictly in psychoanalytic terminology and based them on Freud's theory of female sexuality.

One disadvantage of Zilboorg's work is that he mistook his audience. Psychoanalysts have shown little interest in his work—perhaps because they only seldom meet cases of puerperal breakdown in their practices—and it would be difficult to find a reference to his papers in the psychoanalytical literature. By contrast, non-Freudian psychiatrists have regarded his studies as sufficiently important to warrant detailed scrutiny, but have been faced with the difficulty of having to wrestle with his terminology.

A more intrinsic shortcoming in his work was that, in leaning so heavily on Freud's formations he became involved in certain of the latter's errors (or omissions): firstly, the relative neglect of interpersonal factors consequent upon his discovery of the hitherto unrecognised importance of unconscious fantasy; and, secondly, the masculine bias, characteristic of his era, which led to an unflattering view of female sexuality; to the theory of 'primary penis envy' and a distorted view of the significance of childbirth to the mother.

Leaving aside possible criticisms of Zilboorg's view on the significance of unconscious fantasy in the psychopathology of postpartum breakdown, one can still see that he gives clear clinical evidence to support his assertion that postpartum schizophrenia occurs in women whose history reveals that they have had marked masculine leanings and suffered from serious sexual disharmony—to the extent, in many cases, of complete sexual frigidity. Zilboorg does not, however, leave his thesis at this point, but goes on to compare postpartum schizophrenia with non-puerperal schizophrenia, asserting, amongst other things, that in the former cases the homosexual element tended to be greater and the degree of frigidity less. These comparisons were based on clinical evidence that is not nearly so well documented as that which supports his primary conclusions concerning frigidity, and are theoretically less satisfying, for they imply that he believes postpartum breakdown to have a specific form and aetiology. Several workers, of whom Anderson was the first, have sought to assess the validity of Zilboorg's thesis.

Anderson[5] compared a series of puerperal and nonpuerperal schizophrenias and came to the conclusion that there was no significant difference between the two in their sexual constitution or history of frigidity. However, it is not surprising that he should find a comparable degree of sexual disharmony in the two series, for sexual difficulties, such as homosexual leanings and frigidity, are clearly not related exclusively to the predisposition towards puerperal breakdown, but are personality factors liable to be found in the history of all mentally disturbed women (a fact to be discussed below). Insofar as it was desired to investigate statistically the question as to whether sexual problems play a part in the development of puerperal breakdown—an undertaking that is fraught with methodological hazards—it would have been more appropriate to compare a series of cases of puerperal breakdown with a control group of healthy puerperal mothers, for this would at least have contained the possibility of disproving Zilboorg's main thesis. That this was not done is to be attributed to a confusion in Zilboorg's thinking, and in the thinking of those who have attempted to assess his work, as to the possibility of finding a *specific* aetiological factor in the history of postpartum breakdown.

Frigidity, that is, sexual unresponsiveness, is, as the word implies, an attitude of mind—a coldness, or lack of emotional warmth, felt by the woman toward the man, resulting in a rejection of his advances. The word is sometimes used to apply exclusively to the woman's behaviour in coitus, rather as though such behaviour was separate from the rest of her personality—sometimes, in fact, as though it were a condition of the sexual organs *in vitro*, as it were—but such use of the term is indefensible in view of the fact that frigidity in sexual intercourse occurs only in women whose relationships with men are, usually, characterized by fear, hate, envy, and rejection; in short, in women who cannot love. Moreover, their incapacity to love, although most manifest in their relationship with men, commonly extends to all their human contacts, and the therapist, whether male or female, who undertakes the treatment of such a case, is likely to meet with a persistent rejection of his efforts to approach her.

When such a woman has a baby the probable consequence will be an inability on her part to respond to him with the warmth and love which he requires and clearly yearns for. This does not mean that she will have a puerperal breakdown, but it does mean that she is placed in a position of severe stress: that of having a clear, and even desperate, demand made on her to provide something that she is incapable of providing. Whether she has a breakdown or not will depend not only on the degree of her frigidity but the rigidness of her personality structure, the temperament of the baby, and the environmental setting during the puerperium.

The search for a specific aetiological factor in the personality or history of the woman who has a puerperal breakdown derives its impulse from a failure to appreciate the complexity of the human individual and her existent state. So many factors, past and present, enter into the specific traumatic situation that results in an individual becoming psychologically ill at a particular moment in time that one cannot predict the occurrence of such an illness with any degree of accuracy (cf. Hutten 1956). One can only say that the presence of certain factors makes the development of illness possible or even likely.

I have laboured this point not because I consider Zilboorg's thesis concerning frigidity to be of great importance in itself (it is much too general to be of use in selecting those women who are likely to develop postpartum breakdown), but because the way in which psychological factors have significance in the development of the illness has so often been misconceived. Further research may increase our knowledge of the pre-psychotic personality of these patients but is unlikely to make the prediction of illness possible.

The only known specific aetiological agent in postpartum breakdown is childbirth. This specificity shows itself in the nature of the illness not by any unique formal characteristic, but by the development of particular types of conflict which centre on the fact of childbirth. To the patient and her therapist these conflicts are important, and the fact that certain constellations of conflict have a measure of universality—at least in one particular culture pattern—is worth rec-

Childbirth, the Family, and Breakdown 97

ognizing and charting. The conviction that a specific aetiological agent could be found in the physiological or psychological make-up of the mother has led to a neglect of other factors in her environment (e.g., the setting of the confinement, the innnate temperature of the baby, the nature of her relationship with her family), that could contribute to a breakdown. It would be interesting to know, for instance, whether there is a correlation between breakdown of the mother and a tempestuous disposition in the baby or whether home or hospital confinement is the most likely precursor of psychological disaster.

In order to negotiate successfully a change of circumstance, a person needs to be able both to come to terms with the new element in his life and to maintain meaningful contact with those aspects of his previous existence that continue to remain necessary to his sense of identity. Difficulties arise if the new element is incompatible with previous ones or if his integrative capacity is low.

There are many ways in which such difficulties can beset a parturient mother. In order to contact her baby psychologically (to enter *his* world) she must give him her attention and make accessible to him, and to herself, the relevant areas of her personality. This will be difficult to do if:

a. her repression of her own infantile experiences is very strong;
b. she is not permitted, either by the real demands of others or her compulsive attention to their real or fantasised demands, to concentrate her attention on her baby; or,
c. she has an unrealistic conception of the nature of a healthy mother-baby relationship and/or of her own particular relationship with this particular baby.

The central feature of these adverse factors is the absence of an undisturbed, unprejudiced, realistic perception of the actuality and potentiality of the mother-baby experience. There is interference with her immediate experience of the baby; she is alienated from him and preoccupied with unrealities or irrelevancies. This state of mind constitutes an identity crisis for which there would seem to be three possible modes of resolution:

1. An attempt, in reality, to break through to the full experience of the baby. In this case the presence of the baby stimulates in the mother a recognition of an experience so valuable that she is prepared to wrench

herself away from rigid preconceptions and commit herself to the baby. If this is successful the alienation will dissolve, although other family relationships which have not been prepared for such an event, may suffer. If it is not successful—if the mother miscalculates her strength or circumstances are against her—she may suffer the consequences risked by all those who put themselves in a vulnerable position.
2. Either immediately, or after an abortive attempt at a healthy resolution, the mother may withdraw into a state of illness, in extreme cases to the extent of total alienation from her baby. When this occurs in a family or community which does not understand the real nature of the mother's plight, a vicious circle of interaction takes place between mother and milieu resulting in her further disintegration. This is particularly likely to happen in a rigid, idealized family setting.
3. The mother may consolidate her state of alienation by acting in a way that convinces herself and others that there is neither crisis nor cause for alarm, that, on the contrary, she and the baby are well, happy, and in tune. During infancy, especially if the baby is by nature a quiet one, this may not be a very difficult defence for her to maintain, for his withdrawal can easily pass unnoticed, and manifestations of serious distress can be rationalized as having a physical origin. But it may be the beginning of a malignant process, for the mother is liable to have committed herself to a defensive attitude towards the real nature of her child, and, as the years go by, may become increasingly ruthless in her attempts to suppress evidence that her maternal capacity is in doubt. This reconstruction of a cumulative process between a progressively defensive mother and a psychically crippled child may indicate the kind of path which leads to the fully developed syndrome of the 'over-possessive' mother.

The mother's compulsive need to regard her child as normal and satisfactory derives not only from the necessity to conceal maternal failure but from fear of the disturbing fantasies about him that may have been associated with her original alienation. In respect of such fantasy, it may be useful to consider again the relationship between the mother who breaks down and the one who rears a sick child.

In postpartum breakdown a frequent fantasy of the mother is either that of the immaculate conception of a Christ-child or the production of an ugly and evil creature resulting from intercourse with the Devil. In the former case the mother becomes consumed by a dread of envy, in the latter by shame and guilt; in either case birth is significant as uncovering of what had been previously hidden.

A similarity can often be seen in the preoccupations and anxieties of the mother of the schizophrenic. The determination with which she keeps her child under control, although explicable in terms of her possessiveness, can also be understood as a need to conceal him from the eyes of the world. Not only does she seclude him within her house—a procedure that may symbolize his retention in her womb—but she demolishes his very identity. Moreover, the focal point of intrafamilial discussion is usually the question of public disgrace and the necessity to remain ordinary, respectable members of society. It is as though a monster were being concealed. Such concern could perhaps be thought of as a natural shame in the face of insanity appearing in a family member, but this does not fit the clinical observations. Not only have such fears and behaviour preceded the outbreak of psychosis, but they focus on the moral issues important to the particular culture, on acts such as sexual promiscuity, illegitimacy, rudeness, and so on, liable to be condemned as wicked rather than deemed insane. In fact, psychotic behaviour in the child is often tolerated to a remarkable degree and even encouraged. The reason for the encouragement of bizarre, rather than conventionally unconventional, behaviour may lie in the mother's regarding her child as different—special in the way that Christ was special. But he remains a Christ who is unrevealed. The child, in lieu of a real identity, accepts the only one offered and assimilates its split to his own defence mechanisms. [Note: I would not now be so dogmatic about the nature of a 'schizophrenogenic' mother and the effect of her behaviour on the child.]

One way of formulating the similarity between the premorbid personality of the mother who has a breakdown and of the one who rears a schizophrenic child is to consider both to be in a state of compensated hysteria. According to classical psychoanalytical theory, hysteria in a woman results from a masculine identification based on an envy of the male. As such, it is a dissatisfaction with what she really is, and a desire to be, and to be recognized as, something else. This would seem to fit the clinical facts whether one accepts or not the belief that sexual rivalry is the true origin of the condition rather than its most blatant manifestation in our culture.

An important element in hysteria is the need to prove one's case to the other person; fantasies give insufficient gratification and the object remains important as a source of verification. The hysteric plays her drama before the high court of public opinion, however much she might deceive herself that this is not the case; and is therefore much preoccupied with status, respectability, propaganda, indoctrination, moral issues, and all the power politics that are appropriate to such a situation. Insofar as she is successful, she is not, of course, called a hysteric. In order to avoid defeat she may resort to desperate methods of manipulation such as the assumption of the role of a helpless invalid, or even to simulate insanity, but however degrading some of the positions she may adopt, she never accepts what she feels to be the basic position of inferiority, nor is she able to recognize that the reality of which she is afraid does not condemn her to true inferiority, worthlessness, and meaninglessness. An additional hazard to which she is subject is the fear that if she fails to indoctrinate others then they (assumed by her to be moved by the same motives as herself) will reduce her to a pawn in their own game.

This type of motivation and method is in accord with the behaviour and aim of the mother of the schizophrenic who adopts every means at her command to persuade herself and others of her superior maternal capacity and moral worth.

Although as has been shown by recent studies, the pathogenicity of such families derives from their functioning as a gestalt, it is tempting to think of the mother as the kingpin of the system. Not only would this be more in accord with the psychoanalytical theory of the aetiology of schizophrenia, which gives prominence to the agency of infantile fixation (when the significance of the mother to the child is, of course, paramount), but the impression gained in observing this kind of family is that the brain behind the system of thought is the mother's. Moreover there are reasons for expecting it to be. It is the woman who is most likely to adopt such measures since (a) she is forced into indirect methods of attack and defence owing to the man's greater social power and (b) the myth that she propagates—namely, the importance of family relationships and particularly of maternal care—is one calculated to improve her status.

The woman who thrives on accomplishments of this nature relies on the capacity and readiness of her victim to respond to his cues according to the rules of the game, rules which are derived in part from previous interaction with her. When faced with a stranger, who has neither a conception of nor an immediate capacity to learn the rules, she is in a serious predicament, especially if she cannot escape him nor find a judge who will arbitrate in her favour. Yet this is precisely the situation in which such a woman finds herself immediately after the birth of her baby. In his naïveté he can only cry, but his cries may derange her.

The similarity noted in the prevailing conflicts and defences of mothers who succumb to these two kinds of trouble does not mean that they necessarily form a distinct and exclusive clinical group; it would perhaps be difficult or impossible to distinguish them from several other categories of women, for instance, those who, for psychological reasons, fail to conceive or maintain their pregnancy. The selection of the person to fall ill and the type of illness depends not only on the personality of the mother but the total family organization. What I am suggesting is that the kind of maternal behaviour which contributes to psychological illness in the child arises out of the mother's need to defend herself against the anxieties which lead some women into a state of postpartum breakdown. This, if it be correct, furnishes us with another reason for thinking of postpartum breakdown in terms of the family system, and not merely an unmitigated individual disaster, for the woman who suffers in this way may be attempting to make a creative endeavour which is at odds with the family system of which she is a member. The recognition that relationships can be crucially disturbed by the entrance of a new family member suggests that postpartum breakdown is perhaps best considered as the most spectacular manifestation of a family catastrophe.

Postpartum health is taken for granted and its occurrence passes uncharted but there would seem to be no essential reason why a healthy puerperium could not be as revealing under scrutiny as an unhealthy one. In a study* of the effect of childbirth on the family, degrees of puerperal health in 'normal' families were observed, and I shall describe here an extract from an interview of a family which subsequently enjoyed a puerperium which we regarded as healthy and successful.

When I first called on the Sumner family I knew little about them beyond the fact that the wife was three months pregnant; and they, in turn, had not much idea of our research purposes. As I walked up to the front door a little girl's face appeared at the window and, in response to my wave, she gave me a broad grin. The door was opened by Mrs. Sumner, an attractive, feminine woman, with a shy, embarrassed laugh and a smile as friendly as that of her daughter. She led me into the sitting room and left me there a few minutes with her

---

* This study was undertaken in conjunction with Diana Lomas, under the auspices of the Institute of Psychoanalysis, London, financed by a grant from the Sir Halley Stewart Trust, and made possible by the collaboration of Drs. Ronald and Rhoda Law.

husband, a reserved man with a strong handshake and less mobile features than his wife. He returned to his seat on the couch and observed me in a not unfriendly way, decided that I might like to take my coat off, and offered me a chair. There was little formality. I was left to fix up my tape recorder, feeling that I was, to an extent, being given the run of the place. After I had it ready I discovered that I had forgotten to bring a tape. Husband and wife put forward suggestions to remedy this: he thought of possible shops or neighbours who might supply one; she wondered whether she could help by taking shorthand notes. However, it was decided that I should return home for the tape, a journey involving a delay of three-quarters of an hour; but the family did not seem to mind. Mrs. Sumner expressed concern about my having the bother of an additional journey and said she would have a cup of tea ready for me when I returned. When I returned the family, sprawled around the room, were eating cream buns and drinking tea; the radio was on very loud, playing pop music. I was welcomed and given a bun and tea, and the radio was turned down, but only a little. After I while I had the tape going and the father turned the radio off.

The earlier part of the recording was dominated by the squelching noises made by Janet, their three-year-old daughter, in her difficulty with the cream buns, and her father's amusement at these noises. Janet took an interest in me and offered me buns and things from time to time, but as the interview progressed she became annoyed at 'too much talking,' made an increasing amount of noise with the help of a toy guitar, and finally had an outburst of rage, resolved only by her mother taking her from the room for a while, after which she recovered her humour and offered me more buns. Both parents listened very carefully to the brief account I gave of what I required of them and did their best to serve me well.

I have concentrated on a description of my impression of the atmosphere of this family partly due to lack of the necessary space to give a full account of its history and partly because I think that the former is a more reliable guide to the nature of the puerperal setting than the latter. My experience in the interview was one of ease and friendship; I felt at home, I was not pressed, and I was given sufficient psychological space to move and breathe freely. When the question occurred to me, 'Would I like to be born into this household?' I felt an unhesitating affirmative, despite the fact that I would not be blessed with much in the way of social advantages. This was a calm, relaxed, friendly, receptive, and flexible family, one that was alert to a person's needs and which did not prejudge issues. It manifested many of the qualities which, in chapter 12, I suggest are those characteristic of maternal love. Nothing that I learned from this family in subsequent interviews contradicted my immediate, spontaneous impression, and when I saw the mother a week after she had the baby she glowed with happiness. On that occasion both her mother and mother-in-law were in the house, and the women appeared to be on very friendly terms with each other.

Although I am suggesting that there is a correlation—perhaps a close correlation—between the calm, receptive, and flexible atmosphere of this family and the successful puerperium, I am aware that many questions remain unanswered. For instance, was the baby a quiet, 'good,' and contented one because of his reception or because he had inherited the placidity of his parents? Would the mother have successfully handled a turbulent baby? Is there not perhaps a danger of introducing an unwarranted moral assumption by equating peacefulness with health?

The state in which we found this family was not necessarily either permanent or ideal. It may be that in other circumstances (without the help of the grandmother, for example) Mrs. Sumner would not have been so successful, or that the family will not be able to care for the child at all stages of his development with such good effect. Some of the comments made by the parents suggested an awareness that they had allowed themselves to enter this quiet, placid phase for the purpose of child-rearing, but did not intend to remain therein for ever. One might perhaps think of this state as the family equivalent of that described by Winnicott as *primary maternal preoccupation*.[6]

In spite of reservations I believe we were witness to a puerperium which was not merely successful (in the sense that there was no breakdown) but creative: a joyous, enriching experience had occurred and a new family member had received a fitting welcome. This kind of event must be distinguished from that in which the baby arrives but the experience is lacking; the event may appear to be successful, perhaps even to be taken by the family in its stride, but there is no real fit between mother and baby; he is enrolled in the letter rather than the spirit of the law. This study, together with others reported elsewhere in this volume, point to the futility of searching for a specific factor in the etiology of postpartum breakdown; the more one learns, the more complete the phenomenon appears and the wider our investigations must become.

References

1. Douglas, G. (1963), 'Puerperal Depression and Excessive Compliance with the Mother,' *Brit. J. Med. Psychol.* 36.
2. Hamilton, J.A. (1962), *Postpartum Psychiatric Problems*, Masby, St. Louis, MO.
3. Mayer-Gross, W., E. Slater, and M. Ruth (1960), *Clinical Psychiatry*, Cassell, London.
4. Zilboorg, G. (1928a),'Malignant Psychosis Related to Childbirth,' *Amer. J. Obstetrics and Gynaecology* 2.
5. Zilboorg, G. (1928b), 'Post-Partum Schizophrenias,' *J. Nerv. and Mental Disorders* 68.
6. Zilboorg, G. (1929), 'The Dynamics of Schizophrenic Reactions to Pregnancy and Childbirth,' *Amer. J. Psychiatry* 8.
7. Zilboorg, G. (1933), 'Depressive Reactions to Parenthood,' *Amer. J. Psychiatry* 10.
8. Anderson, E.W. (1933), 'A Study of the Sexual Life in Psychoses Associated with Childbirth,' *J. Mental Science* 79.
9. Winnicott, D.W. (1948), 'Primary Maternal Preoccupation,' *Collected Papers*, Tavistock, London.

7

An Approach to a Family Study of Childbirth[*]

An understanding of what takes place at the time of childbirth would be useful not only to the therapist confronted with postpartum disaster, but to any longitudinal study of personal and family development and to the psychoanalyst who needs to reconstruct the past of his patients as best he can. The conceptions of the event, however, are, so far as I know, limited to the mother-baby interaction. There is no accepted way of thinking about childbirth in terms of the family.

It is with these thoughts in mind that we embarked on an exploratory study of childbirth as a family occurrence. What follows—observations that have emerged from the study—are to be regarded as a first attempt to find an orientation to childbirth as it effects, and is effected by, the family.

The Study [**]

Thirteen families were studied. Ten of them were obtained from the successive bookings for a second confinement in one general practice.

---

[*] This chapter was originally read to the Psychotherapy Section of the Royal Medico-Psychological Society, London 11 May 1966.

[**] This study, made in collaboration with Diana Lomas, under the auspices of the Institute of Psychoanalysis, was made possible by a grant from the Sir Halley Stewart Trust and the cooperation of Drs. Ronald and Rhoda Law.

Only two families approached refused to participate. Although this was not a controlled study, the majority of the families bore some similarity: they came from the same geographical area (a London suburb), were of similar social class (towards the lower end of the middle class), were each having a second baby, and were in good psychological health (if one defines that as having never required the services of a psychiatrist).

The material for the study came primarily from tape-recorded interviews made at fixed, agreed times, impromptu visits that were made from time to time, and the observations of the family's general practitioner. Three routine interviews were made in each case—during pregnancy, soon after birth and when the baby was six months old—but additional visits took place which varied from family to family. As far as was possible the first interview was made with both parents and child together, in order to get a picture of the family as a whole, and by the same interviewer in each case. The interviews were unstructured—that is to say, the families were encouraged to talk about themselves but were not questioned in a routine manner—in the hope of gaining as characteristic an expression of the family atmosphere as we could. It is recognised, however, that the parents inevitably felt themselves to be in the position of test and were liable to present themselves in the best light, a hazard which we attempted to combat by observations of nonverbal behaviour and attention to inflexions of voice when listening to the tape.

During the course of our observations we found ourselves dividing families into two types of which the following, which I shall call the Barton family and the Richards family, are contrasting examples.

The Barton Family

The first visit to this family was made in the evening, when their child (a girl of two years and three months) was in bed. Mr. Barton worked in the CID (Criminal Investigation Department) and the family lived in a large block of police flats, with a long, stiff climb up narrow steps, but the flat itself was quite attractive.

It was the wife who let me in. She was a large, big-boned woman, full of friendly smiles and boisterously talkative. When she told me later that she had been a policewoman, I was not surprised. One could imagine her, in the nicest way, hauling a thug into gaol, but she lacked the feminine softness that makes for easy childbearing. In the interview she did most of the talking and I thought the husband would be overpowered by her but he gradually got going and had his say. Although quiet, he had an assured manner. They were friendly and helpful to me, put me at my ease, gave me freedom and were not afraid of me or defensive towards me. They spoke readily and spontaneously and enjoyed talking (especially the wife), having a direct interest in what they were saying and a wish to communicate it; there was no self-display and little self-justification. Although they checked, now and again, whether they were giving me useful material, they assumed, in the main, that they were.

Mr. and Mrs. Barton, both just over thirty, had been married six years. There had been one miscarriage before their little girl was born. The birth was not an easy one: toxaemia was followed by induction and forceps delivery, the labour taking forty hours in all. But this did not end the wife's troubles, for the baby cried excessively and could not be comforted. 'I got into a terrible state of nerves,' she said, 'I was at the end of my tether.' The husband, who had previously disliked children, and who had been 'talked into having this baby' took over during these crises, nursed the child in his arms, often up all night and nearly asleep at work during the day: 'I felt the baby was safer with me than with her,' he said. Both husband and wife agreed on this point, attributing it to the fact that he had had a kinder and more loving mother than she.

Eventually it was decided to put the baby on the bottle, after which there was relatively little further trouble. We were both just bloody ignorant,' said the husband, 'and we were given bad advice. It was all quite simple really.'

Mr. Barton has grown very fond of his daughter, Mary, and his attitude towards children has completely altered. 'I like all kids now, whatever colour. I wish too I could feel the same about adults.' It seemed that a previous identity, that of a tough policeman, ex-merchant seaman, had been weakened by the event of the birth. His wife, on the other hand, did not like other people's children although she loved her own.

The birth was due in five months time and Mr. Barton planned to take his three weeks leave and look after Mary while his wife was in hospital. Her mother—'a matriarch'—would be prepared to take Mary to her own home, but was unwilling to come and look after her in the

Barton's house. The parents felt this would add to the jealousy of the baby which they anticipated from Mary. This jealousy appeared to constitute their greatest anxiety in connection with the coming event. Mrs. Barton had decided not to feed the new baby, partly because of her difficulty last time and partly to avoid arousing Mary's jealousy.

The Barton's ended the interview discussing the fact that some people seem prepared to leave their babies to cry for hours on end and to be unaware of what a baby really needs. 'I don't think anybody can really be quite sure what is in a baby's mind,' said the husband, 'so you have to act on the idea that the baby feels lonely and afraid, rather than it doesn't.'

In spite of the fact of the open admission of their difficulties in fulfilling their functions as parents (particularly the wife) the Barton's gave the impression of both stability and sensitivity. By their training and outlook they were not the sort of people who would allow themselves to be ruled by their children, but they did not put discipline first, and they remained in touch with the emotional world of the baby. Crying was not something which could be ignored, but, if excessive, was barely tolerable. Although they gave every impression of a sincere and simple love for their child, one felt that they were not 'naturals' for the job. Mrs. Barton knew, by and large, what was needed and wanted to give it, but owing to her temperament and upbringing could not easily achieve her aim. It appeared to the interviewer that there was to be no reason why this united couple could not find each birth an easier process.

Although Mrs. Barton had indicated her keenness to participate in a further interview soon after the birth, it was not until the baby was ten weeks old that she and her husband could find the time. She had again developed toxaemia in late pregnancy, and the second birth, like the first, had not been an easy one. The baby, a boy of eight pounds, ten ounces, seemed to be functioning well but six days after birth he started to vomit and lost weight. The cause, which eventually turned out to be 'a germ,' was not diagnosed for a week or so, during which time Mrs Barton became very anxious and depressed, as, for similar reasons, she had been after Mary was born. Also, as before, the husband commented on the intensity of his wife's disturbance. But this time there was a difference. He did not state, with pride, how he had come to the rescue and nursed the baby himself, and his remarks about his wife's agitated state of mind were put more strongly.

MR. B.: 'I can now understand why the law gives a whole year for a mother to recover during which time it reduces the charge for killing her baby to one of manslaughter. I can see it now. Last time I didn't. I can see it now in my wife, how much childbirth disturbs a woman . . . .'
MRS. B.: 'Oh! I wouldn't have said I was upset. I didn't have time to be.'
MR. B.: 'You didn't know what you were doing, then. That's all I can say.'
MRS. B.: (laughing uneasily, a little embarrassed and perhaps hurt) 'Thank you!'
MR. B.: 'Your greatest fear was losing him, wasn't it?'
MRS. B.: 'Well, I was dreadfully worried he was going to die, yes.'
MR. B.: (with some bitterness) 'And it wouldn't have mattered twopence to me. Not losing the baby. The effect on my wife would worry me to death. And *did* worry me to death. But losing him wouldn't have meant anything at all.'

In this conflict of opinion as to the degree of the wife's disturbance it is difficult to ascertain who is nearer the truth, but the impression gained was that Mr. Barton, in making his point so emphatically and grumpily, was not merely concerned to present the truth but was lodging a complaint about his wife. And, since he did not appear to be concerned with any failure on her part in relation to the two children, it may be that, in her preoccupation and anxiety with the baby, she had (at least, in his eyes) failed *him*. This would account for the tenor of the husband-wife relationship which pervaded this interview; they were, to a degree, alienated. Mr Barton was relatively surly and spoke little, and criticised his wife in a taciturn manner, while the latter spoke much of her children and less of her husband.

As the parents had predicted, Mary did, in fact, show marked signs of jealousy when the baby arrived. Before his appearance in the house she conceived the idea that he did not really belong to her mother, but to 'another lady,' and although the parents attributed this to confusion, it may have derived from a need to deny the mother-baby tie. Thereafter she became depressed and clinging, and whereas, in the past, she had first sought out her father when in need, now only her mother would do.

MRS B.: 'I went through a stage a few weeks ago of regretting we had had a second child. Mary was so upset. She was just terribly, terribly unhappy. Not so much naughty as unhappy. The little things she used to do so willingly she now refused to do. She didn't ever want me to go out of her sight. After I went out in the day with the baby without her she woke up crying in the night. I don't think she knew herself the reason. And it was only me she wanted.'
MR. B.: 'Normally it's me.'
MRS. B. 'Yes, or either of us would do. And she started to wet her pants. I don't

know, she generally was fractious. The only thing I can say is that she was terribly unhappy. Obviously she was put out a bit. We did our best to make her feel that the baby hadn't made any difference to our feeling for her. I began to regret we'd had another baby . . . But she's quite back to normal now. She wants him to get bigger and more interesting.'

Mrs. Barton emphasised the point that Mary felt no aggression towards the baby, but commented that the way she swung toys near his face was disturbing.

The Barton family did not take the new baby in stride. Husband, wife, and the little girl had all suffered, and in their frank way the parents admitted this to the interviewer, being little concerned to present a good image of themselves. In presenting the truth they were respecting each other (and the interviewer) as persons, and this attitude seemed to be in keeping with their attempt to relate to the children as human beings, to discern their inner worlds and meet their psychological needs. Mrs. Barton's account of Mary's unhappiness is an example of her realistic concern, and, in defending her use of the dummy with the baby, she says: 'I know dentists are against it. But I feel the soul is more important than the teeth.' It was clear that, in using the dummy, she had to overcome a great deal of misgiving and criticism from others, but had decided that it was really in his best interest. In other words she responded individually and thoughtfully towards this particular baby's needs, and not by rule of thumb.

This interview (when the baby was ten weeks old), revealed that husband and wife were more harassed than when seen before the birth. Although, compared to most families seen, the atmosphere was relatively lively and stimulating, and the family seemed to be still very much a going concern, there was some evidence of interpersonal stress. The husband spoke at times with some bitterness towards his wife and baby and the wife presented a somewhat forlorn picture of her lonely day-to-day existence. A degree of depression had entered their lives and they had become relatively alienated from each other.

To locate the cause of this alienation with confidence is difficult. The complaints made by various members of the family centre on deprivation of love and attention; they feel lonely, and probably jealous. Mary, presumably due to her mother's preoccupation with the baby, becomes depressed and craves more attention. The wife feels cut off from adult relationship and misses her husband's company. And what of the husband? Why is he embittered and why does he bury himself in his work? One source of love that he has lost, and he openly declares, is that of his daughter; but it is likely that the wife's depressed preoccupation with the baby has hit him also, and that his carping attitude to her and almost triumphant withdrawal into work are sulky reprisals.

When Mary had been born Mr. Barton took over successfully. By so doing he not only supported his wife but he compensated for any feeling of envy or rejection which the birth may have aroused in him. The first baby was a joint project and his status as father (if not as mother) was high. But when the second baby came, although he took considerable time off work to look after Mary and to receive his wife at home afterwards, he no longer was successful in his role, as saviour and tower of strength. The wife, notwithstanding her anxiety over the baby's vomiting was, in her own opinion at least, in better shape to deal with a second child. One wonders whether Mr. Barton's emphasis on his wife's frailty, may have been, to some extent, wishful thinking. Moreover, deprived of the satisfaction of a part similar to that he enjoyed on the previous occasion of birth, he also loses the interest of his daughter. The evidence suggests that Mr. Barton can support his wife in her maternal capacity provided he is enabled to feel an important participant, and that, after the second birth this was not possible, with the consequence that he withdrew from his wife, thereby providing the basis of a vicious circle which could, if not counterbalanced by the positive elements end in a broken relationship. Why was it necessary for this to occur?

The precipitating factor in the Barton Family's predicament would seem to be their anxiety over the baby's crying and frailty. In part this was a measure of their acute perception and acceptance of emotional experience, including infantile anguish. The parents were distressed by the baby's crying and the wife, in particular, became very preoccupied with this (when a visit was made three months later, the baby had been crying a lot over the past few weeks and Mrs. Barton talked about this at length. The interviewer felt obliged to creep about softly and speak in a hushed voice to avoid the risk of disturbing his sleep). It is likely that the mother's anxiety had forced her to focus on the baby to an extent that left her husband and daughter, who were accustomed to receiving her love, relatively deprived.

It is perhaps important to note that the deprivation is relative. In a family such as this one, in which members have a realistic love for each other, a deprivation will occur if the mother becomes excessively preoccupied with a new baby, whereas families unaccustomed to the experience of perceptive love have less to lose. It is perhaps understandable, if not inevitable, that perceptive families will pass through a period of depression, comparable to mourning, in the postpartum period, carrying the risk that members will become permanently alienated from each other.

Follow-up

A visit was made to the Barton's house when the baby was a year old and the family settled in a new house. Unfortunately Mr. Barton (who, it will be remembered, was in the CID) was called out on urgent business right at the start of the interview, but the immediate impression gained was that both he and his wife were happier people than when last seen, a view that was confirmed by Mrs. Barton's subsequent account.

Although Mr. Barton was still working very long hours life had become much easier, largely because the baby was sleeping well, crying little and, in general, no longer a problem. He was now old enough to enjoy watching his sister play. Mary had been disturbed by the move at first, but now delighted in the garden and her new playmates; she had become more independent and no longer clung to her mother's skirts, although remaining more of a mother's girl than before the birth, that is, the withdrawal from her father had been maintained. Mr Barton, however, played with both children when time permitted, and gained great pleasure from his relationship with them.

During the course of the interview Mrs. Barton's basic attitude towards her children again emerged. To her they were individuals who had to be studied. 'I would like to think,' she said, 'that I'd been able to give the baby the benefit of my experience with Mary and to know how to handle him, but it just isn't true. They're quite different. Of course, I learnt how to change nappies and things like that, but in a way I had to start all over again with him.' She sometimes wondered if she was too indulgent. 'If he wants to do something my first thought is: 'why not? And, of course, sometimes it doesn't work and he makes more of a mess than I can stand. But I can't stand him being miserable if I can help it.' It must be emphasised that this was said without any trace of self-righteousness or intellectual detachment. Mrs. Barton was responding to her baby directly and intuitively. But although this was the only way thinkable for her to behave she yearned for the interests of a non-mother existence, fearing she might become a 'cabbage' and have little to offer her husband or her children when they grew older, and she was making tentative plans to combat this trend when it would become feasible to do so.

In sum, the anxious preoccupation with the baby so disturbing to this family would seem to have three sources:

1. A realistic concern with the baby's inner world;
2. A cultural value-system favouring such concern (the Barton's read Dr. Spock); and,
3. A neurotic inability to tolerate the baby's distress. In a nontherapeutic set-up the neurosis could not be explored, but Mrs. Barton's difficult relationship with her own mother, her feeling that she lacked a natural maternal instinct, the psychosomatic problems, the fear of infanticide suggest a neurotic basis. That the concern was not merely a neurotic one, however, is improbable in view of the warm, spontaneous, lively atmosphere revealed by this family. But from whatever source it derived, the Bartons were openly interested in the inner world of their baby.

The Richards Family

The Richards family lived in a semi-detached house in a very long monotonous, treeless row of similar houses, with a view of the gasworks from the front window. Mr. Richards ushered me into the front room, where we were joined by his wife and five-year-old son. Each member of the family had a kind of stodgy, dull, chunky appearance, emanating from the whole demeanour and facial expression, as well as the clothes; their voices, too, were imbued with this quality. Most of the talking was done by the husband, who had a passionate interest in cars and spoke about them at great length; the wife merely echoed his pronouncements. I felt pinned by the husband's talk. Throughout the interview he focused himself on me, occasionally referring to his wife, sometimes glancing in the direction of James. Both parents conveyed, in word and deed, the idea that a child should remain in the background. If James did something to make his presence known, they reprimanded him rather cursorily, and he stopped doing it.

At the beginning of the interview the boy was writing or drawing. He took a friendly interest in me and at one point offered me a piece of paper and pencil in case I wanted to write. I accepted this, but the parents were quick to say that I would not want to write and that the boy himself had better continue doing it. A little after this the boy seemed to want to tell me something, but the parents were speaking and they seemed unaware of his wish. He sat on a chair on his own, sometimes on the floor, playing with bricks for most of the interview. There was no physical contact or gesture of affection between the boy and his parents. On one or two occasions when James spoke, his mother quickly said: 'Don't be a silly boy.' When he expressed a desire to drive the car, the father laughed disparagingly, with the comment: 'Till something else happens'—implying that his interests were short-lived. The boy had no response to the dismissive remarks to which he was subjected.

The manner in which the parents dealt with James was consonent with their assertions about child-rearing in general and their account of James's early days. Mrs. Richards described her determination, on her return from the maternity ward, that the baby was not going to disturb her during the night. 'I came home with the attitude of mind that he wasn't going to wake me up at night, and he didn't!' The father's comment, for the first few months, had been: 'I like him asleep.' He now quoted, with approval, the ward-sister's boast that they cured babies of wanting night feeds within four days. 'He can do without' was a phrase he used several times, indicating that, in his view, the baby's pleasure in any function was not to be considered. Both parents were very smug about their disciplinary achievements and compared favourably with those who had not been so successful in getting their children to conform and be 'good.'

The Richards presented themselves as a 'family-minded' united couple, who devoted themselves to home and children, had similar interests and joint friends, 'I like being at home,' said Mr. Richards, with fervour, 'I would never dream of being away from home at weekends.' They were very scrupulous and self-denying in their concern to care for James. If he had a cold (which was apparently an almost chronic state of his), the parents would not go out to visit their friends, in spite of the fact that the husband's grandmother, who lived in the house, was well able to mind the child.

Amidst much that was repetitious in Mr. Richards presentation, one theme stood out, epitomised in the phrase: 'We are a very lucky family.' After describing their success with James as a baby, his cooperation in feeding and sleeping and his early response to toilet training, which Mr. Richards attributed to their firmness and lack of anxiety, he went on to say: 'We've been very fortunate that way. Between ourselves we've got no difficulties or differences. Right from the start we both knew what we wanted and we seemed to get there. Of course, as I say, we've been very fortunate. We've fallen on our feet ... We've had just what we wanted. We've not had the problems that lots of people have had. . . . If you're the type of person that worries, a family's the last thing you should think of. A comfortable home, a comfortable attitude, you both know what you want, you both agree what you want, you're settled in your minds—then, a family. There's a procedure for this thing. . . . As far as we're concerned, it's just gone as it should.'

It was surprising to learn, in the face of Mr. Richards's assertions, that this family had in fact suffered a tragedy. Their second child had died, a few years ago, suddenly and unexpectedly, from a respiratory infection. This event, which they described briefly, was referred to as a 'setback.'

Towards the end of the interview the father described himself as 'a bit of a diplomat.' It was necessary for him, he said, to have a happy home and he would keep the home happy at all costs, even if it meant telling white lies. 'I would not want to come home if the place was unhappy.' I know my other home would then be the pub. We've tried to get contentment.'

As the interview progressed I found myself feeling more inhibited and overwhelmed by frustration. These parents were friendly and kind towards me—they gave me tea and insisted on completing the interview even though (I happened to know) they had a pressing engagement—but they prevented me from any form of self-expression. I felt quite unable to make any meaningful comment on anything they said, and found myself wondering what it must be like to grow up in such an atmosphere, as James had done.

The main characteristic of the Richards family was their rigid solidarity, based on the affirmation of traditional values and the denial of tragic experience. They had established a mode of existence designed to avoid trouble and to maintain the status quo, and their method of achieving this goal was not the shrinking and timid withdrawal from life of the overtly anxious parent, but an assertive and positive one. In psychoanalytic thinking it could be considered as a kind of counterphobic measure, but this would be to view it as entirely a negative manoeuvre. Certainly, much of it appeared to be negative and sterile and conducted at enormous cost in terms of spontaneity, imagination, physical pleasure, genuine love, and individual growth. But something had been created, however limited. The defence was not a brittle one and the family functioned in society independently and without shame.

An apparent contrast, however, exists between the selfless devotion of the parents to their child and their lack of concern for his emotional experience. It would seem that the care which the parents provide is based to a large extent on their preconceptions about his needs, and may, in part, be designed to put them in a strong moral position as parents. In such a position they are better able to impose the disciplinary measures on which they so much rely. As we speculated on what is likely to happen when the new baby arrived, we could reasonably forecast that this family, inside their well-prepared fortifications, would soon have the baby organised into their system with the minimum of disturbance to their regime.

Shortly after the birth, Mr. Richards rang up to arrange an interview, but later cancelled it because the baby was in hospital with pyloric stenosis. He was very apologetic about this, and as soon as the baby was out of hospital he arranged an immediate interview. Despite the crisis of the baby's illness and operation, the whole family appeared in better shape than when seen before, and the mother and boy showed more animation. The interview began as follows:

INTERVIEWER:	'Would you like to tell me about events?'
MR. R.:	'The last week has been a long week.'
INTERVIEWER:	'Yes, I'm sure it has.'
MR. R.:	'But apart from that we've finished building the car.'
MRS. R.:	'And you've been in hospital.'
MR. R.:	'Yes, I've had a hernia operation.'
JAMES:	[Interrupting] 'The baby's been in hospital, too. . . . '
MR. R.:	[Ignoring the interruption] 'Did I tell you about that? I knew I was going to have to. I was just on the general waiting list.'
JAMES:	'Do you know, the . . . '
MR. R.:	' . . . but it flared up some. . . . '

The father continued with his account of his hospitalisation and then went back to the subject of his car. During this time the baby could be heard crying in another room. It was left to the interviewer to reintroduce the subject of the childbirth and the baby.

The birth had taken place at home (much against the husband's wishes) because no hospital was available, and was a normal one. Mr.

Richards took two days off work, and Mrs. Richards's mother came to stay and help for several weeks. In spite of Mrs. Richards determination to discipline him quickly, the mother found herself being 'less hard' than she had been with James. The baby fed vigorously, by breast and bottle, but after a fortnight began projectile vomiting. Pyloric stenosis was diagnosed, and an operation was performed from which he made a quick recovery. Since then he had been well, but sleepy, and it had not been possible to restore his routine.

The paradox presented by this family was sharpened by this interview. The kind of defences they had used before were still in operation. One would expect that a family which had already lost one child would have found the baby's illness a terrifying experience, but the Richards appeared to have taken it in stride. At the time of the interview the baby was only just out of hospital, but it was some time before this event was talked about; the main explicit aim of the parents in relation to the baby was still to organise him in a way conducive to peace and quiet; and experience was reduced to the mechanics of life, the times and amount of feeds, and so on. But there was a mellowness and warmth that had not been noticeable before; the commonsensical and unfussed way this family had dealt with the birth and the emergency was impressive, and the manner in which the mother fondled her baby towards the end of the interview was a natural and loving one.

There would seem to be two (interconnected) reasons for this contradiction. First, the fact of successful birth had made them more relaxed and open, more able to give, both to each other and to the interviewer. Their defences against anxiety and tragedy took the form of a hardness and rigidity that saw them through stresses and crises, but these defences were not necessarily always present. Secondly, one of their defences was to present themselves as capable and independent, thus concealing from the interviewer the warmth of which they were capable, but which they feared might be regarded as weakness. Having passed the test of birth (the test relevant to their relationship with the interviewer) and become used to him, they could afford to be more open. That they could now act in this way does not, of course, negate the existence of the defences described earlier, but it helped us to understand why a family so apparently lacking in spontaneous love could live together without showing more evidence of suffering.

The main impression left by the Richards family was of their marked ability to adapt themselves to trouble. They took trouble by the throat, as it were, and ground it into the dust. This capacity enabled them to maintain a stable family life in the face of all hazards and to provide a secure ground for their children. The promptitude with which they tackled their problems did not entirely strangulate emotional life but restricted it to a degree which impressed the interviewers and others who have listened to the tapes.

The birth was dealt with in their characteristic way. Preparations were made, and the baby and his illness were quickly and competently brought under control. Although there was no overt anxiety before the event nor obvious rejoicing afterwards, the family showed, in the demeanour of each member, a decrease of tension and an increase of happiness and well-being. It was an event with positive significance for the family as a unit, and the gain in ease and freedom (perhaps particularly for James, upon whom parental pressure was diminished) outweighed any pressures from added responsibility and jealousies. Insofar as the aim of these parents was the achievement, for whatever motive, of a 'family,' they had had a success and made up for a failure. Insofar as they were relatively insensitive to infantile distress (and their attitude to the baby's crying suggests a rather high degree of insensitivity), they were immune from a traumatic experience which so often undermines parental confidence in the postpartum period. Over the next year the family settled down to a quiet, uneventful, and unreflective existence. Group solidarity and mutual loyalty remained as impressive as ever but life was not a searching quest, and the continued dreariness of their voices suggested the price of this limitation. Although the new baby was given more room to manoeuvre than James had been, the parents appeared to lack the imaginative capacity to enter his world.

Two Contrasting Attitudes to Childbirth

The two family patterns described were not unique in the series and exemplify contrasting types of response to childbirth.

The Barton family was characterised by (1) a warm and lively atmosphere in which a serious if not always successful attempt was being made to understand the personal individuality of the child, (2) an inability to tolerate a baby's crying and a need to do something about it, (3) the possibility of expressed disagreement between husband and wife, (4) a difficulty on the part of the mother in limiting herself to maternity and an inability to breast-feed successfully, (5) an existent but ambivalent relationship between the wife and her mother, (6) a capacity to verbalise easily, and (7) anxiety, problems of jealousy, and husband-wife alienation after the birth; recovery within the course of a year or so.

That a family concerned to make a realistic accommodation to birth which is difficult for them should suffer a period of disruption of the kind described is not an unexpected finding. And perhaps it is not surprising that neurotic and realistic wishes towards the baby should act together in ways that make the mother vulnerable (what makes us hesitant to recognise this occurrence is our tendency to *contrast* neurotic and realistic aspiration and to regard them as automatically in opposition to each other). The problems presented to the family which chooses the course of tuning in to the baby are to some extent similar, whether the reasons for so doing are realistic or neurotic. It requires a degree of preoccupation with the baby which threatens the stability of other interfamilial relationships and an emotional flexibility which may be disturbing and fatiguing to the mother. A possible consequence of this is that feelings of deprivation and jealousy may arise, disrupting the husband-wife and, in the case of a second baby, the mother-child relationship. It seemed, further, that, in such circumstances the elder child could become preoccupied with the mother-baby set-up to such an extent that a previously valuable father-child relationship was in hazard. The depression from which the mother suffered was related to the fatigue, anxiety, guilt, and anger engendered by her attempt not only to please the baby but to protect the others from deprivation as well as preserve some degree of freedom of individuality of her own.

In a situation such as this the balance between success and failure may easily be tipped. The mother has the chief role and it is necessary either that she have sufficient inner security to survive the crisis or that she be 'held' by others. Although fairly secure as a person, Mrs. Barton doubted her maternal capacity and lacked the happy relationship with her mother which could have given her support. Had her neurotic compulsion to adapt to her baby's needs been greater she may well have succumbed to a postpartum depression requiring psychiatric help. But her depression may have been to some extent a necessary accompaniment to a creative change, a measure of her perception of the distance between the baby's need and her ability to meet it, a disillusioning perception without which there could be no internal growth.

The Richards family, by contrast, expected the *baby* to make the necessary accommodation. Although this attitude was most explicit in the Richards family, it was present in several others and showed itself in various ways—in the first place, in the manner of dealing with the baby's crying. In these families the parents, whether or not troubled by crying, let the baby cry and did not pick him up to comfort him. They acted in this way believing that the baby must be cured of this troublesome habit. In one case we have recorded evidence that the baby was left to cry until in a deeply disturbed and (to those who have listened to the tape) disturbing state. What is a psychology that lies behind this attitude?

Assuming that a baby's cry has the biological function of communicating distress to the mother so that she will help and comfort him, one would expect that a mother would naturally respond to it. In these families the response is somehow killed; the baby is thought to be 'naughty,' to be trying to get something (physical handling) that is not his due; and those who do respond to his pleas are regarded as misguided and weak. The baby's viewpoint is, in a sense, invalidated: his needs are not, according to this belief, what he thinks they are or how he presents them. The imputation of such dishonesty in a newborn baby is not in keeping with the limited degree of intelligence which the baby is estimated to have over other matters, and would seem to originate in an unrealistic fear on the part of the parents: the baby, if not broken in at an early age will get out of hand and control the family ruthlessly. The existence of such an underlying fear is supported, in the case of the Richards family, by the parents' attitude towards the discipline of the older child: he must be good, polite, conform, he must be 'made' or 'driven' to do this or that; at all costs he must not become a teenage delinquent. What is of significance here is the emphasis. It is not merely that these parents believe in discipline; they are preoccupied with it to the exclusion of other matters. This preoccupation is in keeping with their social conformity; they are not prescribing one law for the child and another for themselves, for their own lives are subject to the same control and limitation. Their philosophy excludes exuberance, abandon, excitement.

Whether the limitation of possibilities demanded by this approach to life is necessary or desirable depends upon one's sociological, philosophical, and religious beliefs; the psychotherapist would likely regard it as not only unnecessarily crippling and painful but productive of a degree of repression which may lead to psychiatric disorder in later life. Factors suggesting that it is a neurotic, defensive attitude include the obsessive preoccupation with the problem, the amount of anxiety attached to possible failure to achieve the desired placid and calm equilibrium (less manifest in the Richards family than in some other 'conforming' families we observed), the need to justify, and the inability to perceive emotional reality. It appears as less a considered judgement, a sagacious limitation of attention and exploration, than a frightened, compulsive, and rigid withdrawal from the mainsprings of life.

The disadvantages of this kind of family system are offset by certain gains. The kind of pitfalls with which the Bartons were confronted are avoided. The Richards family gave the impression of a solidity and stoicism which would ride crises. It would survive and although individuality be restricted each member knew where he or she stood, a state of affairs which may counterbalance much restriction of emotional searching. Although the Richards's experience of life was not on a level of emotional insight which a psychotherapist would be likely to recommend, one might perhaps be on uncertain ground in assuming that they were less happy or more in danger of psychological disaster than the Bartons. The hazards are different. Because disillusionment is avoided by deliberate limitation of aims, the postpartum depression which can occur in women who idealise their maternal capacity[1] is avoided; the depression is of a chronic low-grade variety characterised by stoical resignation and limitation of experience, easily passing for normality.

There is one sense in which the attitudes of both families towards their babies have more in common than is apparent, and this centres on their neurotic fear of infantile experience. Those who fear primitive emotion may, when faced with a baby like the Richards, deny the significance of the baby's feelings and exert early disciplinary measures. But another way of dealing with their anxiety is to assuage infantile distress as soon as possible; to get it out of the way.[2] In such a family the mother, far from leaving her baby to cry, will hasten towards him at the first squeak and the whole family will go about on tiptoe. Both approaches differ from the realistic and calm appreciation of the baby's needs possible for a mother who is not so overwhelmed by her anxiety that she cannot perceive him.

Conclusions

Perhaps because we entered these families with no problem on which to focus and with no questionnaire—indeed, with as little organised perception as we could manage—it was the general atmosphere which most impressed us. We found that this atmosphere, which made its impact in the first few minutes, and which we thought of in such terms as warm or cold, receptive or constricting, manifested itself in all aspects of the family including that which we had come to study, that is, the attitude to childbirth. Many studies find their framework either from long established formulations or from the requirements of the investigation itself. But these—certainly the latter—are not necessarily the most appropriate. It may be that the most meaningful aspect of a phenomenon to study is that which makes most spontaneous impact. This would amount to saying that leaving aside the genetic constitution of the baby, the most important factor in the birth, both from the point of view of the baby, and for the subsequent family adaptation, is the atmosphere into which he or she is born—the overall reception which a newcomer is given.

Inevitably it is difficult, if not impossible, to decide whether a classification one makes is chiefly a function of the phenomena under investigation or the mental set of the observer. It can, perhaps, only be judged pragmatically. The classification which emerges from our study hinges on the contrast between those families able to observe, make room for, and allow expression to another person in their midst, and those which prejudge and control his activity. Over the course of the first year or so these two types of families were subject to differing hazards, some of which we have attempted to delineate.

It is perhaps worth noting that the attitude of mind of the Richards-type family towards the baby is markedly nearer to that of the 'schizophrenogenic' family towards the offspring[3] than that of the Barton-type. If this observation is correct, it suggests that the anxiety, depression, and disharmony characteristic of the latter's early experience may be the price paid in overt suffering for the sake of future mental health of the baby.

Postscript 1997

In a paper written in 1985, Joan Raphael-Leff[4] based her study of mothering on 'clinical insight, observations, and questionnaire data.' She postulates a model 'delineating two basic orientations towards mothering: the 'facilitator' who 'adapts to her baby, spontaneously interpreting his/her needs' and the 'regulator' who 'promotes the baby's adaptation by establishing a routine and regulated predictability.' Raphael-Leff's study was more systematic and less descriptive than the study reported above, and focused on mother-baby relationships rather than on the family as a whole; yet it is surprising (or should it be?) that the dichotomy she postulates is in many ways so similar to the one that we found ourselves making.

Raphael-Leff observes that: 'The Facilitator embraces pregnancy and motherhood as self-realisation, the high point of her feminine identity. She believes that babies are sociable from the start, aware of their own needs and able to communicate these. She intends to dedicate herself to facilitating her child's well-being in the first years of life by *adapting* herself to the baby, empathically interpreting and spontaneously meeting his/her every wish. The Regulator views infants as pre-social and sees her maternal task as socialization—regulating the baby's behaviour and training him/her to fit into a realistic routine. She feels this task may be shared with other caretakers. Mothering to her is an interchangeable role she engages in, whereas to the Facilitator it is an exclusive way of life.'

The defences with which the two types of mothers try to circumvent their vulnerabilities are different. Whereas 'at-risk regulators' use 'exaggerated control, rigidity, and denial'; 'at-risk facilitators' use 'idealisation, over-identification, and altruistic surrender.' We would say that, in Raphael-Leff's terms, Mrs. Barton was a facilitator-at-risk and Mrs. Richards was a regulator-at-risk. We would, however, wish to emphasise firstly, that an understanding of the mother-baby relationship depends, in no small way, on an understanding of the family as a whole, and secondly, that although we hope that classifications of the kind used in this chapter can be helpful they may also be used to oversimplify a very complex phenomenon.

References

1. Lomas, P.(1960), 'Defensive Organisation and Puerperal Breakdown,' *Brit. J. Med. Psychol.* 33, p. 61.
2. Szasz, T.S. (1959), 'The Communication of Distress between Mother and Child,' *Brit. J. Med. Psychol.* 32, p. 161.
3. Wynne, L.C., I.M. Ryckoff, J. Day, and S.I. Hirsch (1958), 'Pseudomutuality in the Family Relations of Schizophrenia,' *Psychiatry* 21, p. 205.
4. Raphael-Leff, J. (1985), 'Facilitators and Regulators: Vulnerability to Postnatal Disturbance,' *Journal of Psychosomatic Obstetrics and Gynaecology* 4, p. 151.

8

Observations on the Psychotherapy of Puerperal Breakdown

Introduction

While on the staff of the Cassel Hospital, Richmond, I had the opportunity of working with several mothers who had broken down in the postpartum period. In this chapter I shall describe in some detail the psychotherapy of two of these cases, discuss the roles of the therapist and of the hospital, and attempt to formulate some of the goals which would seem to be within the reach of treatment.

The mothers were treated as inpatients and were encouraged to bring their babies with them—an offer which most of them accepted. Others, being quite unable to tolerate the presence of their babies, declined at first, but brought them in as treatment progressed. One or two never achieved this reunion. In some cases husbands also came to the hospital for week-ends. Owing to the environment in which these patients were treated, acute, unmanageable psychosis had to be excluded. Treatment was by individual psychotherapy based on psychoanalytic principles.

Puerperal breakdown is not a well-defined clinical entity. The illnesses of these mothers fell into a variety of categories from the point of view of descriptive psychiatry: depression (either neurotic or psychotic), schizophrenia, hysteria, anxiety state, and mixtures of these

---

Published in the *British Journal of Medical Psychology*, 34, 245 (1961).

syndromes. Cutting across these classifications was an interpersonal pathology: a disturbance of the mother-child relationship to an extent that was damaging to the child (if not so obviously to the mother). In short, these mothers could look after their babies either very unreliably or not at all.

Case 1

Mrs. R. was admitted to the Cassel Hospital with her eleven-month-old baby boy. Although she had never been psychiatrically ill before, she became acutely confused three days after the childbirth, with the result that she was sent to a mental hospital and given a course of electroconvulsive therapy (ECT). On returning home she continued to act and talk in a strange way and was unable to tackle her household duties though she managed to look after the baby. She had a further course of ECT without gaining improvement and, a few weeks before her admission to the Cassel Hospital, ran away from home in the middle of the night wearing her husband's clothes and having cropped her hair.

Her general practitioner, who was concerned at her manifestly psychotic behaviour, had advised her against bringing the baby to hospital, but in spite of this she arrived at the Cassel Hospital with the baby and an unspoken demand that he be accepted too.

Her appearance was striking. She was a good-looking woman whose close-cropped hair and staring, dreamy eyes made one think of Joan of Arc. During sessions she talked for the most part like a playful, teasing child, and much of her inconsequential chatter displayed primary-process thinking. Among these thoughts were references to men, whom she despised and hated, to frightening machines, to 'big dams bursting,' and self-accusations for 'stealing knives,' for not being feminine, for not washing her hands, and for not loving her baby or her husband. She took a delight in quoting verses of Edward Lear and Lewis Carroll—in particular, Old Father William who stands on his head 'although I fear it might injure the brain, but now I am perfectly sure I have none, why I do it again and again.' Often her quotations could be seen to be slyly malicious comments about the (male) therapist.

In complete contrast to her usual irresponsible chatter she talked of her baby, Timothy, with sanity and with real feeling and was quite obviously devoted to him.

In the hospital she was encouraged, in common with the other mothers, to look after the baby and this she did with the utmost care and patience. Timothy was her life and she had little time or capacity to attend to anything else. She was very indulgent towards him and allowed him to make a dreadful mess. In this she identified with him, for she herself was extremely untidy, although not to the extent of being dirty. It was also noticeable how she and the baby looked like each other. There were no rows between them, he never was known to cry, and everyone agreed that he was a singularly beautiful baby, even though he was rarely responsive.

During sessions her hate and contempt of men became more blatant. 'I'll tell you a tale that I told to another patient who believed it,' she said, with gleeful mockery. 'I told her that I was a Mormon who had six husbands. I went shopping on a Yak and my chief husband walked behind. I left the other five at home to do the washing up.' She aroused in the therapist a tendency to treat her as an irritating yet amusingly mad child who needed humouring. Before long she spotted his reaction and it became clear from her associations that she resented it. The interpretation was made that she needed to be such a foolish and mad child because she was terrified of being taken seriously, yet felt bitterly angry that she had to act in such a way. Her anger caused her to be all the more foolish and confusing in order to induce a similar despair in the therapist. This interpretation was, unlike nearly all others made, listened to seriously and acted upon, and she became more coherent afterwards.

She was clearly very proud of Timothy, but at first reluctant to admit this. Later she said 'I think he is perfect and other mothers' babies are . . . ,' leaving the sentence unfinished. 'But it is not good form to go strutting about the place.' It seemed that all her hopes and ideals, especially her masculine wishes, had been projected on to the baby, perhaps to delusional intensity, and that she had surrendered her life masochistically to him. This sacrifice of herself went as far as relinquishing her social claims and adult status, as though she felt that if she were not taken seriously then she would be allowed to enjoy the baby. This masochistic surrender was unstable, for she felt vicious hatred towards males, and in order to avoid feeling hate towards her baby she made her main target her husband and, later, the therapist. The figures of her childhood remained colourless and unreal, particularly that of her mother. Her father she described as 'stuffy and pompous,' yet she obviously admired him. She was the middle of three sisters, felt that her parents would have preferred a boy, and greatly envied her elder 'brilliant' sister. However, it seemed particularly difficult for her to relate interpretations in a meaningful way to her childhood, and at most she would feel diffusely that she had been unloved and misunderstood, but could not remember this in any detail. It also became gradually clearer how, in spite of the satisfaction derived from her baby, she felt desperately empty and unwanted. 'I don't know why I came, or why I come' she said. 'I can't go home. My husband wouldn't let me.' (This was not overtly true). Her intense envy of men became clearer, and she began to talk of her actual problems with her husband; of how she used to play a major part in the financial affairs of the family because she was so much more efficient than him, but now she can't do it, nor can she drive the car; of how lucky he is, like all men, how pompous, how useless. She became upset at the thought that their sexual life was unsatisfactory, and berated the therapist for not helping them.

After she had been at hospital five months she attempted suicide by taking aspirin tablets. For several days prior to this she had been depressed, but the actual precipitating cause was a rebuff by the therapist who made a mistake over her session time. Her suicidal attempt brought the response of real, yet angry concern on the part of the staff and she expressed her anger in return. In the following session the therapist also expressed both anger and concern. The suicidal attempt was interpreted as an attack on the therapist due to feeling rejected, a means of finding out if he was really concerned about her, and a desperate attempt to convey to him how ill she was—in the only way she could. The impression gained was that she was pleased by, and grateful for, our reaction to her suicidal attempt.

Following this episode there was a considerable clinical improvement. She looked better, took part, often quite prominently, in social activities and even went out for one or two evenings to enjoy herself, leaving someone else to look after Timothy. There was also a change in Timothy, who began to show signs of aggression for the first time.

Soon after this she learnt that her younger sister had given birth to an illegitimate child, and commented briefly on not having been told of this and on her parents' unsympathetic treatment of her sister. She therefore went to visit her sister and identified herself closely with her, recalling her own feelings of shame at the time of childbirth. Indeed, it seemed to be a feeling of shame which had hitherto prevented her from talking about the childbirth and puerperium. She felt ashamed of her failure to stand up to the test and bitter towards her medical attendants for not having enabled her to do so. In recalling these experiences she said: 'I'm no good as a woman. I'm not fit to be a mother.'

At this point, unfortunately I was due to leave the hospital staff, and during the final phase of the relationship her aggression towards me reached its maximum. My date of departure was delayed by a month, and this the patient could not tolerate because she felt it was being done to confuse her. Her fear of being confused was discussed and she became very angry. This time, however, she expressed he anger openly, demanded an immediate change of therapist (to a woman) and stormed out of the session. Following this, her paranoid fears of being confused diminished and she reported in the next session that she no longer believed particular magazines were deliberately put in the waiting room in order to upset her. She was also able to talk for the first time about her feelings of anger towards Timothy. 'I am afraid of terrifying him,' she said, 'but perhaps he is tougher than I think.' This seemed to be a reaction to experiencing that I was tougher than she thought and could take her direct expression of anger in the previous session.

The decision was made that she would remain in hospital in the care of another therapist, and although it was feared that this might totally disrupt the improvement hitherto made, the transition proved to be less traumatic than had been expected. This was perhaps due to close collaboration between the therapists, to the support of the hospital environment, to her relationship with the sisters and other patients, and to the continuing success of the mother-child set-up. She gradually became more realistic, able to recognize the therapist as a separate being with his own life to lead, and she returned home eighteen months after admission. We felt a certain amount of concern for the development of her child because of the intensity of the mutual identification and lack of overt aggression between them.

Owing to this patient's relative inability to discuss her early life, and to her confused state during the following childbirth, it has not been possible to make a very satisfactory reconstruction of her psychopathology. The essential features of her illness, insofar as they were understood, would seem to be as follows. Although never mentally ill up to the time of the childbirth she could not have been described as well-adjusted; in her own eyes she was an outsider, a wayward person, a kind of tramp, and a permanent misfit. Her chief defence had been a detached and ironically playful attitude to life, which she had never taken quite seriously. She had not made a satisfactory sexual adjustment, having too great a masculine identification and envy of men.

Childbirth proved to be a painful and humiliating process, and in retrospect she angrily berated her medical advisers, particularly her doctor, at the same time maintaining that they were very kind. It was at this crisis in her life that her detached, yet organised attitude to the world had broken down, and her rage emerged in a dissociated way—directed primarily towards men. It seems likely that childbirth caused her envy and hate of men to reach breaking point, because she experienced it as a castration. A consequence of this was her desperate attempt to reassert her masculinity by cropping her hair and dressing as a man.

It is not sufficient to describe her experience of childbirth as a castration, in the sense of a loss of masculinity, for her resultant feeling was one of complete emptiness and loss of her sense of identity. That loss of identity (or, subjectively, of 'ego-feeling') is the essential feature of schizophrenia has been suggested by Federn[1], and more recently by Freeman, Cameron, and McGhie[2]. According to Erikson, although castration becomes a more sufficient term if the fantasy of 'body-phallus' is present—as it was in Mrs. R.'s case—the sense of identity involves more than the awareness of the body, and is intimately related to the ego-ideal.[3] Mrs. R.'s picture of herself had collapsed utterly under the impact of childbirth and she felt bitterly ashamed.

Lynd[4] has called attention to the close relationship between feelings of shame and loss of identity. She describes shame as the loss of trust in expectations of oneself and of other persons, as opposed to guilt which is a transgression of a code. As an example of shame she cites the feelings of a small child who had carefully planned a surprise present for a loved adult who failed to appreciate it. Similar experiences are the lot of a mother who has idealized her baby, and Winnicott[5] has described the feeling of disillusionment in the new-born baby as being an important factor in the mother's hate for the child.

Mrs. R. acted out these feelings symbolically by bringing pathetically messy and more or less illegible 'essays' (representing her genital, her baby, and her confused self) to the therapist and being very interested in what he thought of them.

Mrs. R. was a mother but nothing else. In becoming this she was no doubt responding to a biological urge, but was also compensating for her loss of ego-feeling by identification with the baby who was idealized. This relationship was the thread by which she maintained her hold on reality, and the baby served the purpose of a transitional object or fetish. The willingness to sacrifice herself for the child is in keeping with the schizophrenic's willingness to sacrifice maturity and social development for the fulfilment of a primitive wish. A mother with a character disorder is often faced at childbirth with the unhappy choice of either maintaining her defences, at the expense of a failure of empathy with the baby, or a pathological breakdown of defences in an attempt to feel empathy. Mrs R. chose the latter, if choice it can be called. As the disruption of personality was not such as to break up the mother-child relationship entirely, she found it easier than most women to be an indulgent mother and could allow her baby to make such a mess as would have driven another mother crazy. There were, however, disadvantages in her maternal capacities. Owing to the intense identification it was difficult for the baby to develop a personality of his own; he even looked remarkably like her. Moreover, owing to her own lack of aggressiveness, he did not learn (or dare) to be aggressive himself. In spite of her idealization of the baby, her relationship with him was on a much more mature level than were her dealings with others, and she showed real love and concern for him.

In her relationship with the therapist she showed a mixture of identification and rejection. Her transference was that of the psychotic who has a desperate hunger for objects with whom to identify, coupled with an acute sensitivity to any lack of interest, and a tendency to reject the object angrily and violently. Perhaps the greatest demand made by this patient was to be recognised, and it was following recognition, or interpretation concerning recognition, that clinical improvement occurred. It was very important indeed for her that her baby was recognized, but that was not enough. She needed to be recognized herself. What this patient seemed to be doing, following the loss of identity imposed on her by childbirth, was attempting to establish a true sense of self by being recognised as a real person while at the same time maintaining some sort of pseudo-identity by identifying herself in an unrealistic way with the baby, the therapist, and the hospital.

Case 2

Several years earlier, Mrs E., now thirty-one, had developed acute anxiety about her duties as a midwife and had become a drug addict. Her first child, a girl now two years old, had been in a residential nursery since a few months old when the patient had resorted to drugs to an extent considered dangerous to the child, and had herself been admitted to a mental hospital. Mrs. E. was referred to us from the mental hospital when she was seven months pregnant with her second child, because the referrer felt she might stand a better chance of keeping her baby if she came to the Cassel Hospital after her confinement.

After a normal confinement in a maternity hospital she went home, and at first felt there was no need for her to come to hospital. Soon, however, she became acutely anxious, found the responsibility of her house and the baby boy to be more than she could bear and asked to be admitted.

Mrs. E., slight and quietly feminine, came to the first interview in a state of profound depression and sat meek and passive, as though waiting for judgement to be passed on her. When, after encouragement, she began to speak, it was of her feeling of utter uselessness as a wife and mother, her fears of the responsibility for the baby and her doubts as to whether she and the baby would be able to fit in with hospital life. She remained in this depressed state throughout the fortnight's assessment period, and the therapist, affected by her intense feeling of helplessness and the knowledge of her addiction to drugs, felt very doubtful of the wisdom of attempting to keep mother and baby together.

It soon appeared that some of her despair derived from the fact that she felt quite sure we would not keep her on for treatment and would assuredly send her back to the mental hospital, regarding her as unfit to look after her baby. She also knew that she had no chance of looking after the child on her own at home, and would, in her anxiety, again resort to drugs. When it was agreed that she should stay on as a patient, together with her baby, she showed great relief and gratitude, and from that moment her demeanour changed. The therapist's fears that an improvement based merely on another's belief in her maternal capacity would not be maintained by such a sick patient were gradually allayed as she began to show a great determination to sort herself out, as well as a pursuit of truth that is rather rare.

The main theme of interpretation was that she had repressed most of her aggression towards her possessive mother (and more recently her husband who organized her household activities as though she were a child) and that this was now hidden behind a masochistic need to placate others and abase herself. It gradually became possible to show her this in the transference. She had an enormous respect for doctors, and treated the therapist as though he were a god, attempting to please him in every way, but this was in part an aggressive attitude, for she thereby concealed herself from him and deprived him of an alive and human relationship with a real person. Following this understanding her tense and reserved demeanour during sessions slowly became replaced by an increase in directness of emotional expression towards the therapist. Although her earnest cooperation still contained an element of conformity, she had a genuine urge to recover which made real work possible.

Mrs. E.'s self-destructive flight into drug-taking (which had made her unable to look after her first baby) had not only been an escape from responsibility, but also a surrender of her own life and her own wishes to other people whom she compelled to deprive her and discipline her. This masochistic urge had caused her to act in such a way that she was sent to a mental hospital, leaving her baby in the hands of her mother. This act was a condensation of her need to surrender her most loved possession to her mother (whom she had always felt was envious of her) and a revengeful desire to attack her mother (and the world in general) by ridding herself of the anxiety-causing child with whom she was identified, and leaving the burden of this care to others. In taking her into hospital with her baby we had not only, by implication, shown our belief in her as a mother, but in her lovableness as a child. Unlike her, we were unafraid of infantile anxiety and hate. This now enabled her to look after her own baby.

The envy which Mrs. E. feared from her mother was based not only on a projection of her own feelings of hate and envy, but on historical fact. Her mother, a most dissatisfied woman, had contracted an unhappy marriage which ended in divorce when the patient was fifteen. Even as a child the patient remembers feeling sorry for her mother, who cut a rather pathetic figure in her attempt to remain young to keep pace with her, and who was terrified of ageing. Mrs. E. had grown up afraid of her own femininity, afraid to tell her mother when she first became engaged, and when she was first pregnant. She was afraid, too, of showing her feminine capacities and of asserting herself as the woman of the house towards a husband who took on domestic responsibility and acted rather like the woman of the house himself.

Mrs. E., although inwardly angry about being deprived of her function had never before been able to assert herself in this way. Now she began to do so. She became more forcible in her marital relationship, and took to going home on the weekends and controlling domestic affairs. She was no longer awed by her husband's managerial capacities. While in hospital she looked after her baby conscientiously and well, although tending to worry excessively about his health and being unable to take an open pleasure and pride in him. One major source of her distress was the shame and guilt she felt about her failure with her first child who remained in the residential nursery and whom she visited occasionally. She would break into tears when talking of her. The interpretation was made that she was identified with this baby girl whom she had needed to destroy, just as she had now masochistically destroyed her own life. A few months after her treatment began she decided that she had become capable of looking after the little girl and that she wished to do so. She took her from the residential nursery and brought her to stay at the hospital. This girl was backward, probably because of her long motherless stay in an institution. She was withdrawn and presented an immense therapeutic problem to the mother who, however, responded with patience and understanding.

As treatment continued she showed increasing assertion towards the therapist and began to fear that he was possessively using her for his own ends. This could be seen as a repetition of her feelings towards her mother. The feeling that she was being constricted by the therapist's own needs, and her desperate desire to be free and to be herself, represented a recurring theme which was the crucial one in her therapy. Because of this the decision of when she would go home was left as far as possible in her hands, and she made it without hesitation at the end of ten months' treatment. Whether this was wise is perhaps difficult to say, for serious sexual difficulties had not been resolved, and her decision to stop treatment undoubtedly contained a defensive element. Nevertheless, it was felt that her capacity for real maternal feeling had been established, and that this decision to return home was an expression of it.

Discussion of the Case Histories

The two cases described above showed marked differences in psychopathology and symptomatology (as indeed did all the cases in this series) but certain similarities can be seen. Both women had been unsure of their femininity before childbirth and both despaired of their maternal capacity afterwards, feeling themselves to be incapable of loving their babies. Neither woman could tolerate her baby's aggression. Although they bother reacted differently to it, these mothers had much shame and first-aid measures were needed to counteract it. The only way to do this was by showing belief in them as mothers. This was done by taking them, with their babies, into hospital, where they received not only encouragement in their function of mothering but protection against their own violent feelings. When this need was met, individual therapy based on psychoanalytic principles became possible.

The Function of the Hospital

Bringing the puerperal mother into hospital together with her baby—a therapeutic manoeuvre described by Douglas[6]—could be seen to have the following effects on the mother:

1. She felt believed in as a woman and as a mother and she felt that her child was believed in.
2. Any unconscious guilt she felt for bearing a child was relieved by the permissiveness of the hospital, which played a parental role.
3. She felt protected from her own hostile impulses towards the baby (engendered by unconscious factors which will not be dealt with here).
4. She could escape from the hostility and envy which, rightly or wrongly, she feared from her relatives, particularly women.
5. She was eased from the burden of looking after her husband, a burden which several of these patients, owing to pathological husband-wife relationships, felt to be excessive.
6. The hospital gave her the support which even a 'normal' puerperal mother, in her state of mental disorganisation and reorganisation, requires of her environment.

One disadvantage of bringing a puerperal mother into hospital is the consequent disruption of important family relationships. This was prevented as far as possible in our series by allowing mothers who had older children to bring them into hospital and by encouraging husbands to visit whenever they could, and in some cases to live at the hospital, if only for weekends. It seems likely that less sick mothers with good family relationships could satisfactorily and perhaps more profitably be treated as outpatients.

The effects of hospitalization described above could be expected, to some extent, as a consequence of taking the mother and child into a hospital. However, the hospital setting in which these cases were studied was particularly orientated towards mothers and children.[7] The mothers were treated not as sick and helpless patients, but as responsible people free to conduct their own affairs and have a say in hospital management, especially as far as arrangements for mothers and babies were concerned. Within this culture-pattern the mothers could feel that it was taken for granted that they would be able to look after their children. There was no atmosphere of compulsion which those mothers in revolt against maternity as a symbol of feminine subjection or parental demands would resent. Moreover, each patient had a hospital Sister allotted to her to whom she could turn as a woman and mother-substitute. Opportunities for relationships with other mothers were plentiful.

The atmosphere provided is in striking contrast to that to which most mothers who are confined in hospital are exposed during the puerperium. This is not to suggest that the present-day maternity ward is the cause of the puerperal breakdown, but in many of the mothers described (all of whom had hospital confinements) it was undoubtedly a contributory factor.

The Function of the Therapist

The role of the therapist cannot be entirely separated from that of the hospital, for although his function is primarily to interpret the patient's psychopathology, he is a member of the hospital staff. He decides, with the help of his colleagues, whether the patient will be taken on for treatment. By his tolerant attitude and his belief in the patient, he supplies her with the essential support previously described. His role as interpreter is also bound up with this function.

It is difficult to define a psychotherapeutic technique for the specific treatment of puerperal breakdown as it eludes clear definition as a clinical entity. However, it is perhaps useful to set down the tentative theoretical approach developed as a result of treating these mothers, and to describe some recurrent psychopathological themes which required interpretation.

Puerperal breakdown is a pathological reaction to new psychological experiences which are associated with childbirth. These experiences include changes in the body image, close contact with a primitive human being with whom identification is made, and alterations in other personal relationships, especially those of the family. This produces an identity crisis characterized by a breakdown of the previous mental organisation, both adaptive and defensive, and the need to make a new adaptation. In puerperal breakdown, owing to faulty emotional development in the mother and/or an unsatisfactory environment during the puerperium, this new adaptation cannot be made, resulting in anxiety, confusion, and the production of pathological defence mechanisms.

The following factors are important in producing this outcome (and require interpretation during therapy):

1. The mother's identification of the baby's crying with her own primitive aggression, causing her to hate and reject him, and setting in motion a vicious circle of hate and guilt[8];
2. Dissatisfaction with the feminine role, causing her either to reject maternity or to identify it with a phallic performance, thereby incurring feelings of guilt;
3. Fear of the envy of others for her successful creative act, for its social significance, for its unconscious meaning in terms of oedipal strivings, and the vicarious pleasure it brings in terms of primitive infantile enjoyment of life. Such fear of envy is augmented if the baby is idealized;
4. Masochistic tendencies designed to ward off the envy of others and to counterbalance feelings of guilt.

The Aims of Pyschotherapy

In thinking about puerperal breakdown it is necessary to decide whether one needs (a) to treat a sick mother who has symptoms which must be cured, after which she may or may not be able to look after her baby, or (b) to treat a relationship, namely the mother-baby unit, which has gone wrong. These patients were approached with the belief that the latter view is the more correct one.

It follows that the first and immediate aim of psychotherapy must be to help the mother over her crisis with the hope that she will be able to continue her function as a mother. This can be best done by giving her a suitable and stable environment in which she feels allowed and encouraged to be a mother, and by interpreting the most urgent anxieties connected with her possession of the baby. If this can be achieved quickly the vital mother-baby link can be maintained, and in many cases maternal feelings will emerge. It is important to decide, in the case of extremely sick mothers, whether the baby's only hope of psychological survival is temporary or permanent separation of the partners. The dangers in making this decision lie in the fact that powerful emotions deriving from unconscious sources and affecting both doctor and patient may influence the result. However, by far the greatest danger lies in underestimating the mother's capacity if she is given a chance to reveal it.

Once the crisis is over, and the patient is able to look after her child, the main question is at what point to be satisfied with her recovery. The patients in our series could be divided into three classes from the point of view of outcome:

1. Those mothers who made a quick and stable recovery, their personalities returning to the state prior to childbirth, with its accompanying defence mechanisms—a result which gives immediate satisfaction but may lack prophylactic value;
2. More severely ill patients, particularly those characterised by almost complete frigidity and intense envy of men, whose personality problems had been more clearly revealed by the childbirth, and who remained, despite all efforts at therapy, bitter and unhappy women. It usually became possible for such patients to return home and to look after their families, but life remained essentially without meaning for them;
3. In some cases, either because the mother did not respond quickly and return to her normal equilibrium or because the disturbance had caused her to become dissatisfied with aspects of her personality, further psychotherapy was attempted. Following breakdown of defences, these could be reorganised in a different way. In mothers of this kind a real change in personality structure took place which showed itself both in the transference situation and in a changed pattern of family and social relationships.

Acknowledgments

I wish to thank Dr. T. F. Main for his help and encouragement with this work and Dr. J. Davie for supplying some of the clinical material.

References

1. Federn, P. (1952), *Ego Psychology and the Psychoses*, Basic Books, New York.
2. Freeman, T., J.L. Cameron, and A. McGhie (1958), *Chronic Schizophrenia*, Tavistock, London.
3. Erikson, G. (1956), 'The Problem of Ego Identity,' *J. Amer. Psychoanalytical Assoc.* 4, p. 56.
4. Lynd, Helen M. (1958), *On Shame and the Search for Identity*, Routledge & Kegan Paul, London.
5. Winnicott, D. (1958), 'Hate in the Countertransference,' in *Collected Papers*, Tavistock, London.
6. Douglas, G. (1956), 'Psychotic Mothers,' *The Lancet* 1, p. 124.
7. Main, T.F. (1958), 'Mothers with Children in a Psychiatric Hospital,' *The Lancet* 2, p. 845.
8. Szasz, T.S. (1959), 'The Communication of Distress between Child and Parent,' *Brit. J. Med. Psychol.* 32, p. 161.

9

Puerperal Breakdown and Defensive Organisation

In normal pregnancy psychical changes occur in the mother which can be thought of as a change in 'ego-feeling' (in the sense used by Federn) in the direction of greater 'bodilyness' and a shift of interest from 'outer' to 'inner.' These changes do not constitute a withdrawal from reality, for the mother is concerned with the reality of the fetus and is preparing herself for the primitive contact with the baby when he is born. The psychical changes require an ability to permit a partial disintegration of the previously established psychical organisation, the admission into consciousness of new perceptions and the reestablishment of a new organisation. None of which occur readily in those who have a rigid defensive organisation.

At childbirth the ordinary mother is involved in a further psychical change by the 'orgasm' of parturition, followed by the complex state described by Winnicott[1] as 'primary maternal pre-occupation,' in which she achieves the empathy with the baby so vital for his healthy development. These events necessitate flexibility on her part, for she has to relax her defences against the primitive urges which the baby now demonstrates so uncompromisingly and openly.

Although in this condition the mother usually shows regressive features, in particular a dependent need to be 'held' by a protective

---

This is a revised version of a paper published by the *British Journal of Medical Psychology* (1960) 33, p. 61.

environment, she also normally possesses a mature sense of responsibility and concern. The risk of further regression is, however, always present. The ego, in its undefended condition, is potentially vulnerable to a traumatic influx of unconscious impulses, as well as to the demands of the super-ego and an external reality which may be particularly demanding at this time. (In this chapter I am concerned with the intrinsic vulnerability of some mothers rather than any failure to hold her at the time of birth and afterwards).

The Breakdown of the Defensive System at Childbirth

Many mothers, particularly those who use the mechanism of denial, are able to maintain or increase their defences during pregnancy. In this way they survive it without overt difficulty, but later succumb to a traumatic breakthrough of impulses when the baby has arrived. Unlike those who gradually achieve a state of undefendedness during pregnancy, such a mother has rigidly held out against this change until the intensity of the neonate's biological claim on her attention proves too great.

The mothers in this series did in fact suffer from character disorders. Intense problems relating to sexuality and aggression (most of them were sexually frigid) were contained by a rigid defensive system. The character traits most in evidence were those involving moral masochism and the mechanism of denial. It was rare for a mother to have sought psychiatric help previously.

The attitude these mothers took towards their present illness was revealing. They were either desperately (and often dramatically) trying to maintain their defensive systems and to avoid hospitalization, or they were equally desperately seeking it. Some mothers were in an acute and confused state of indecision about this. Others seemed to fear that if they ever relaxed their defensive guard they would fall into a dangerously regressed state. A few did in fact become excessively dependent while in hospital, although never unmanageably so.

Mrs. A. is a mother who sought to maintain her previously rigid defensive system and in whom the mechanism of denial was of special importance.

Aged twenty-five, she was admitted with her ten-month-old baby girl. She complained of anxiety attacks, breathlessness, and headaches

Puerperal Breakdown and Defensive Organisation   143

which had started a few weeks after the birth of her baby. However, she gave the impression to the Hospital Sister, who made a visit to her home prior to admission, that she herself did not seek treatment and was only coming to hospital to please her husband.

She was an attractive woman who responded quickly with a bright smile but who when alone or thoughtful looked depressed, wan, and uneasy. She very quickly brushed aside all problems and was at pains to show how 'normal' she was. For instance, while admitting that she was more or less frigid she added 'but so many women are like that, aren't they? It's all a matter of time and settling down.' The question of whether she had any trouble with the baby was majestically swept aside: 'It's not as though I were one of those women who know nothing about it; I have had experience of babies before [referring to her sister's].' Her description of her relatives did not give a picture of real people. She denied all problems of childhood, believing her own to have been only happy and uneventful and her parents to have been consistently good to her. She was able, however, to express some jealousy about her older sister and younger brother. The only point at which she showed emotion in describing her past history was when she spoke of not being able to go to university.

In her own eyes she had always been a mentally stable person. She was somewhat inclined to worry about her health, and in the past three years had developed a fear of cancer. She had paid frequent visits to her doctor, asking him to inspect lumps on her tongue, bones and elsewhere, but was never reassured for long. She was quite sure that she did actually have more lumps and abnormalities than was usual. She consistently denied that her anxiety was disproportionate, saying: 'Any woman would be the same. One is always being told these days to go to your doctor and make sure.'

She felt her marriage to be successful although she had been unable to have intercourse for the first year and even now experienced no pleasure in it. She was the dominant partner in the marriage and organized everything; there were never any rows.

During her pregnancy she felt especially well and happy and (unlike most women) denied any misgivings about her confinement, which went well and easily. Her only complaint while in the maternity hospital was that insufficient notice was taken of the baby. Soon after she returned home, however, she experienced anxiety, breathlessness, headaches, and paralysis of her limbs, which usually occurred when she was alone with the baby. She also developed a breast abscess. One particularly severe attack of anxiety came on when she was returning to hospital for her postnatal examination.

Between the beginning of her illness and her admission to the Cassel Hospital, her father had died rather suddenly. She was genuinely distressed about this—it was one of the rare occasions when she had allowed herself real feeling—but this event does not appear to have played an important role in the etiology of her illness.

Her life was organized with a puritanical attitude to relaxation and pleasure, and one severe anxiety attack which occurred in hospital was brought on by a party during which she allowed herself to 'let go' more than usual.

In treatment, her defences, particularly denial of anxiety and feeling, diminished to some extent. She was able to reveal a haunting fantasy of her baby lying with a knife in his stomach, but she was unable to let herself be aware of any feelings of hate towards the baby. Although the baby was 'good' and quiet, she was very afraid of *his* aggression. She said 'these days one has to be a good mother in order to stop the child growing into a juvenile delinquent.' The impression gained was that the baby was felt to be good but full of pent-up aggression. Indeed, he represented a picture of her own mental state, and this provoked death wishes towards him. She became anxious not only on account of the revelation to the world of her true turbulent self in the shape of the baby, but also because she directed against him her own violent superego reaction to hostility.

Thus there was danger of her inner conflict between primitive urges and super-ego being replaced by an outer war, the child representing for her, her own aggression. This conflict had manifested itself internally in the past by her fear of cancerous lumps (a symptom representing a condensation of her phallic aggressive wishes as well as her need for punishment).

Like almost all cases of puerperal breakdown, Mrs. A. consciously desired her baby (several of the patients in this series were longing for more babies even during their illness). In her case this seemed to be not so much a mature wish as a need to keep a 'good object' intact and to fight off inner persecution.

In general, the fears of what would be revealed by the real externalization of the baby could be seen in the mothers of this series to be of two kinds. First, fear of the 'badness' projected onto the infant, resulting in shame and anxiety over the baby's aggression. Secondly, fear and guilt about their pride at the success and pleasure represented by the baby, and mobilizing a need for punishment.

The outstanding character trait of another patient, Mrs. B., was moral masochism. She came from a very religious family in which any expression of joy in life was regarded as emanating from the Devil. Humility and suffering, particularly in women, were regarded as virtues. The patient was the youngest child, and had two brothers. When she was five her father, whom she had loved, left home and she never overcame an intense feeling of bitterness towards him, a feeling which she displaced on to all men. Her relationship with her mother was a chilly one. When she grew up she left her own country, came to England and married a man who was sick, unreliable, and socially her inferior, yet whom she could serve and succour in her masochistic way. It was clear that she despised him, but she gained satisfaction from the feeling of spiritual superiority deriving from the relationship.

She conceived in order to please him, but during her pregnancy became tormented by fears that the baby would look like her father-in-law, a man she loathed on account of his uncouthness and uneducated manner of speech.

To her dismay the child turned out to be a boy. She soon became terrified lest she should kill him, and she was admitted in a confused state to a mental hospital when the baby was four months old. She remained there for several months, being given electroconvulsive treatment, and when discharged refused to return to her husband and baby. Eventually she was admitted to the Cassel Hospital in a withdrawn and depressed state. She proved a very difficult patient to treat, remaining sullen and withdrawn, silently expressing intense bitterness and suffering.

Her mother-in-law willingly took care of the baby. Mrs. B. continued to see her child and husband at weekends, in spite of the fact that she no longer concealed her hate and contempt for Mr. B. Then, surprisingly, she conceived again. Outwardly she was horrified at this 'mistake' but one had the impression that she gained a secret satisfaction from it. The same sequence of events occurred as in her first pregnancy. She became obsessed with the fear that this new baby would be coarse and uncouth like her father-in-law. Her resistance to interpretations was very strong but it gradually became possible to understand some of the meaning of her obsession. The uncouth baby stood not only for the hated male but also for her own repressed lively and primitive instincts which in her childhood had been considered so sinful. Her attempts to deny the physical existence of the fetus and of the 'dirty' instinctive act that had produced it led her to fantasies of an immaculate conception. She came to regard the psychotherapist, rather patronisingly, as a 'physical doctor' and although by now she had given up her religious beliefs, sought guidance and blessing from a priest.

In a desperate attempt to deny the exposure of her supposedly 'evil' self in the form of the baby, she constructed an intense idealization of him. She also increased her masochistic and paranoid defences in order to avoid guilt-feelings, and so organised things that the therapist was plagued by a variety of social agencies (and even her embassy) who were concerned at her pitiable sufferings. In view of the fact that another complete breakdown was feared during the puerperium these defences were analyzed as far as possible. Her anxiety mounted as the time of her confinement approached, but she had her baby and looked after her satisfactorily, although she would not return to her husband and the other child and went instead to live with a woman friend. It is difficult to estimate what bearing psychotherapy and hospital support had on this relatively satisfactory outcome of what had appeared to be a disastrous state of affairs, for the fact that the second baby was a girl was undoubtedly important.

Like Mrs. A., her tendency in pregnancy was to increase the defences by methods of denial and idealization, but she was less successful in her attempts at denial.

In both cases the defensive systems, though intensified during pregnancy, broke down during the puerperium, with consequent intense anxiety. Mrs. A. was more able than Mrs. B. to deny her anxiety and feelings of hate, for her defensive system, although rigid and vulnerable, was more stable. Through the development of a moral masochistic character Mrs. B. had managed to deal with life without mental illness up to the time of childbirth. At that point this character mechanism broke down and the hate and anxiety which it had previously bound came into the open.

Socarides has suggested that the clinical picture of moral masochism has three essential stages.[4] First, 'compensated masochistic adaptation' in which an uneasy truce exists between defence and adaptation, fear and rage being quiescent. Secondly, 'decompensated masochistic adaptation' marked by 'fear, rage, urgent pleas for fulfilment of love needs, and the sudden eruption of defensive manoeuvres.' Thirdly, there sometimes follows 'masochistic adaptive failure,' which may result in suicide or violent outbursts against the lost love object. He states 'decompensation' appears when the struggle for love, the reassurance against and fending off of the fear of abandonment has become a losing battle. Self-punishment is an effort to relieve guilt, to demonstrate one's harmlessness and goodness, and thereby to retrieve the lost love object.'

This way of looking at moral masochism is helpful in understanding the effects of childbirth on a mother such as Mrs. B., who, before breakdown, was in a state of 'compensated masochistic adaptation. Childbirth, involving the loss of the idealized object in the shape of the baby, and the revelation of badness and sin, brought about a decompensation with its resulting anxiety, rage, and guilt.

Moral masochism and denial are similar manoeuvres, both being concerned with rigid control and the concealment of aggression. When the aggression becomes externalized in the shape of a baby, who can represent either repressed or repressing forces, the mother's defences do not function successfully and she becomes consumed with anxiety. This is, inter alia, what happened in the two cases described.

The Psychodynamics of the Breakdown

The hazards faced at the time of childbirth by a woman with a rigid defensive organisation can be viewed in several different ways:

1. The inevitable biological state of undefendedness against inner and outer forces involves a risk of a pathological collapse of defensive organization with appearance of anxiety and symptoms.
2. The mother with an impoverished ego and a rigid defensive system is specially dependent on the possession of what Melanie Klein refers to as a 'good internal object.' During pregnancy 'ego-feeling' is enhanced by her new internal possession and all that it represents, but at childbirth she has to relinquish this narcissistic gain in order to love the baby instead of herself. Because of her relative incapacity for real object relationships she cannot easily love her now external baby, as an external object and to reestablish her narcissistic equilibrium.[2] Moreover, as during pregnancy the baby was felt to be an idealized inner object, she will be disillusioned by the *real* baby and by his reception. This disappointment in herself and in her world may result in a loss of her sense of identity.

3. The transposition of the baby into the outer world is particularly hazardous for mothers whose defensive systems are concerned with concealment. This applies especially to those with problems of exhibitionism, as well as to masochistic women. The baby who now appears before the world (and herself) symbolizes not only all her concealed primitive aggressiveness for which she expects punishment, but may equally represent all her buried hopes, pleasures, and ambitions which in turn evokes an anticipation of the envy and jealousy of others.

Various Methods of Solution

The outcome of childbirth for a mother with a character disorder of the type discussed will vary according to the relative importance of various factors concerning both inner conflict and environmental circumstances:

a. Her defensive organisation may be traumatically disrupted. The resultant anxiety is then dealt with by a pathological reorganisation of her defences, varying with the individual, and resulting in neurosis or psychosis. This constitutes puerperal breakdown.
b. She may be able to maintain her defensive system. In this case the baby, although outside, remains idealized and unreal. The extent to which this matters in very early stages of mothering is debatable, but it may later only lead to the child not being allowed to have an individuality of his own.
c. In favourable circumstances the mother may be able to use the breakdown of her defence mechanisms to establish herself as a new person more in touch with her real life. In these cases the baby can, in one sense, be thought of as a psychotherapist whose interventions are not so harsh and untimely as those made by the babies of the unfortunate mothers who break down.

Conclusion

The therapeutic study of patients with postpartum breakdown suggests that the woman with a particular type of character disorder is in danger of mental illness during the puerperium. Prominent among the reasons for this is the challenge offered to a rigid defensive system by the need to own, and to relate to, a child who is bound to remind the mother of her own primitive and repressed wishes. Such elements as the use of denial and moral masochism, which are concerned with concealment, are particularly vulnerable to the revelation which the act of childbirth implies.

Acknowledgements

I wish to express my thanks to Dr. T. F. Main for his help and encouragement in this work, and to Dr. B. Zeitlyn for supplying some of the clinical material used in this study.

References

1. Winnicott, D. W. (1956), 'Primary Maternal Preoccupation,' in *Collected Papers*, (1958), Tavistock, London.
2. Payne, S. (1936), 'A Concept of Femininity,' *Brit. J. Med. Psychol.* 15, pp. 18–33.
3. Socarides, C.W. (1958), 'The Function of Moral Masochism: With Special Reference to the Defence Processes,' *Int. J. Psychoanal.* 39, pp. 587–98.

10

Dread of Envy as an Etiological Factor in Puerperal Breakdown

Introduction

In the last chapter I discussed the conflicts faced by the mother who had up to the time of childbirth successfully used the mechanism of denial. One particular conflict mentioned was the fear of envy aroused in the mother who idealised her baby. Here I shall go into more detail about the part played by a dread of envy in the aetiology of puerperal breakdown in susceptible cases.

During pregnancy and childbirth a woman is required to make changes in her defensive organisation in order to meet the challenge presented to her by close contact with the primitive drives of her baby, and during this time she needs to be 'held' by her environment. The most suitable person to perform this service for her is her own mother, from whom she has experienced mothering, who can serve as a guide and teacher, and with whom she can identify in order to stabilize her threatened sense of identity during this crisis. It is not surprising therefore that the custom in most societies is for an expectant mother to seek the aid of her own mother or of an elder woman who can act as a mother-substitute. This state of affairs can only be satisfactory, however, if she has had a good enough relationship with her mother for her now to be able to entrust herself to the care of a mother-figure

---

Published in the *British Journal of Medical Psychology* 33, 105 (1960).

with a feeling of confidence. If her relationship has been one in which feelings of hate and envy predominated she will either be unable to avail herself of this support or will do so with fear and mistrust.[1]

Nearly all the patients studied in this series had manifestly poor relationships with their mothers and were unhappy in childhood. The most usual family pattern was that of a father who had been physically absent or psychologically ineffective, and a mother who had been lonely, bitter, possessive and envious. In some cases this picture was convincing as a historical fact; in others it was coloured by a projection on the parents of the patient's own bitter and envious feelings. These mothers were neither able to gain support from their own mothers during childbirth nor could they believe in their own maternal capacity. One factor in this situation could be seen to be fear of their own mother's envy of their creative achievement.

Case 1

Mrs. J. was a meek woman of twenty-four with a pale and harassed face and a childish manner and voice. She was an only child whose father had died when she was seven, and whose mother, in her grief, had taken to drink and left her alone in the house for long periods. All her life she had felt inferior and was easily embarrassed on social occasions, a symptom which could be seen to be the result of repressed exhibitionistic tendencies. She remembers once as a child having paraded naked through the fields, and had always wanted to become a ballet dancer. Prior to her illness she had never regarded herself as neurotic, and had been happily married for two years; her husband was in the Forces and she only saw him on weekends. She remained well during her pregnancy and confinement, but a few days after the birth of her boy she became depressed and began to feel that things were unreal. Her mother looked after her for the first fortnight after her return home from the maternity hospital. Although her relationship with her mother was not an easy one, she felt that she had received some support from her and she only broke down after her mother left her. She had no relatives living nearby and no neighbours upon whose help she could draw. She became confused and anxious, her main symptom being a feeling that she did not know the time or the date of the baby's birth, and that he was not really there at all. She was admitted to a mental hospital, but after a few days she secured her

Dread of Envy as an Etiological Factor in Puerperal Breakdown 153

discharge although feeling no better, for she longed to be reunited with her baby. Because of this she was subsequently admitted to the Cassel Hospital with her baby when he was a month old. Although rather frightened at the idea of coming to hospital again, she welcomed it as a refuge. One of the facts which emerged during therapy was that she was unable to feel that she possessed the baby herself, on account of fear of the envy of others, particularly her mother. She liked to be effusive and loving towards the baby but simply could not be so when her mother was present. She pretended to be uninterested in the child, and let her mother take him over. She similarly deferred to her husband, who also had maternal tendencies. This depreciation of her baby, to the extent of hardly recognizing his existence, could also be seen as deriving from a denial of her lifelong exhibitionistic wishes. The baby stood for all that she longed to be and wished to display yet had to conceal.

The origin of her confusion about the date of birth and of her feeling that the baby was not really there lay in a need to pretend that her very successful exhibitionistic act of childbirth had not really occurred.

During the course of psychotherapy she became able to understand some of this and also to express bitter anger at having to be so masochistic. On one occasion in particular, she experienced a paroxysm of rage and shame, and sobbed helplessly throughout the session. Following this she became more able to stand up for herself, especially towards her husband. It could now be seen why the hospital regimen, by which she had been encouraged to look after her baby in her own way, and to have full rights over him, had been of such great and immediate help to her.

After she left hospital, and while attending a few sessions as an outpatient, she reported a remarkable change in her attitude to baby, husband, and mother. She now felt the baby belonged to her and she could speak of him with pride, saying, 'I know he's real now. You should feel the weight of him.' She had also developed a healthy attitude of nonchalance towards the constant advice about the baby given by her mother and her husband. 'I'm quite happy to let them talk,' she said, 'but I go my own way now.'

Case 2

Mrs. D. was a woman of twenty-seven with two children, a son aged two-and-a-half and a daughter aged seven months. She came into hospital with the girl only, as her problem was that she could not tolerate the boy, whom she had sent away from home because of his vomiting and crying. Since his birth she had been in constant fear that she would injure him in one of her outbursts of rage against him.

She was herself illegitimate and had been brought up by her mother and rather Victorian grandmother in an atmosphere where men and sex were regarded with repugnance. As a child she was unable to express her feelings and could only cry when alone. She was unable to speak to her mother about her first menstruation and concealed her developing breasts with shame.

In the treatment situation all of this was repeated. She regarded herself as a burden to the therapist, without the rights of other patients, and was in constant fear of being discharged for being troublesome. She greatly envied another patient's capacity to cry bitterly in the sessions and was amazed that this patient was not thrown out for such behaviour. It became clear that she felt herself to be unwanted, a shame and a nuisance to her therapist (mother). It also became clear that she regarded the boy in the same light and was identified with him. She had great difficulty in bringing him to the hospital at first, and she could not tolerate his making a noise because as she said, 'It calls attention to myself.' It was only after some months that she became aware that she really liked him to be 'tough and masculine,' and she and the therapist came to understand that he represented herself as she would like to be—lively, noisy, dirty, and all that she felt herself not allowed to be. He was male, as she too wanted to be. Thus she projected her masculine wishes on to him, gaining a secret pleasure from this, but openly condemning him. Moreover, she blamed herself for his shortcomings but was quite unable to accept credit for any admirable qualities in either of her children.

A very important cause of her condemnation of both herself and her boy was found to be a fear of her mother's envy if she herself became a successful mother. She was unable to show any liveliness or enthusiasm towards her children in the presence of her mother, and organized things in such a way as to give her mother a feeling of superiority and the ability to win the children's affection, handing over the care of

Dread of Envy as an Etiological Factor in Puerperal Breakdown 155

them to her on the slightest excuse. In the case of the boy her behaviour was in part due to a need to rid herself of a troublesome being with whom she was identified, but she also needed to surrender her children masochistically to her mother and really yearned for encouragement and permission to keep them. In the hospital setting, with permission to keep and look after her children, and with the help of interpretation of this problem as it showed itself in the transference, she also brought her boy into hospital. After a year's treatment she was able to take both children home and look after them herself, but she never became able to feel real pleasure in her son.

Although some of her fear of the envy of her mother could be seen to derive from a projection on to her mother of her own greedy and deprived self, the main factor seemed to be that her mother was in reality a lonely, bitter, and deprived woman, who had failed to keep her man and had never achieved the capacity for mother-love. Because of this the patient could not bear to hurt or provoke her by herself being successful as a woman and as a mother.

Case 3

Mrs. B. was a young woman of twenty, whose first baby was a girl. Pregnancy for her was a blissful state until the last month when delivery came within sight. A few weeks after the birth she made an attempt to gas herself after giving her child to the neighbours, and was admitted to hospital. She lived in terror of the envy of other women towards her baby and had obsessive thoughts that she ought to give the baby away. This method of dealing with fears of envy by sacrificing her possessions was a characteristic one and she recalled how as a child she had always given away her chocolates and sweets.

The woman she most feared was her mother-in-law, a very possessive widow who lived nearby and came each day to take possession of the baby, while Mrs. B., unable to defend herself, stood by in silent rage and despair. Clearly the hospital was for her a sanctuary. She also feared the envy of her elder sister who had always acted maternally towards her, and who was herself married but apparently sterile. An improvement in Mrs B.'s condition occurred when she received the news, while having treatment, that her sister had at last succeeded in conceiving.

In contrast to most of our other cases, Mrs. B. presented no great therapeutic problem. With the support in her maternal capacity given by the hospital culture and by achieving some insight into her fears she quickly regained her previous happy (albeit slightly hypomanic) personality.

Case 4

Mrs. D., a woman of thirty-one, had been a drug addict for many years. She was one of the few cases who had sought psychiatric help prior to having her baby. However the fact that she had first resorted to drugs because of anxiety over her duties as a midwife suggested that childbirth represented a special emotional problem to her.

When her first child, a girl now aged two, was nine months old, her own mother came to stay with her. She felt that her mother considered her unfit to look after the baby and within a few days resorted to drug taking, which resulted in her admission to a mental hospital, leaving her mother in possession of the little girl. This child was eventually sent to a residential nursery.

Mrs. D. subsequently spent her time in and out of mental hospital, and became pregnant again. It was now arranged that she come to the Cassel Hospital with her baby after the confinement with a view to attempting to keep mother and baby together.

In appearance she was a good-looking woman, but withdrawn. During the first few diagnostic interviews her dejection was so profound that, knowing that she was a drug addict, I felt quite hopeless about her, and had doubts about putting into operation the planned attempt to keep mother and baby together. However, the attempt was made, and from then on the patient's demeanour changed and she gradually came out of her depression. She later revealed that she had felt quite hopeless about looking after the baby on her own at home, and yet had wanted to keep him more than anything else in the world. She had not been able to express this at the time, but it seemed that what she had most needed was for someone to believe in and permit her maternal capacities.

During therapy she began to realise that her mother (whose husband had left her when the patient was a child) had always attempted to appear much younger than she really was, and had discouraged the patient from going to dances because she had been envious of her daughter's youth and femininity. The patient recalled her difficulty in

Dread of Envy as an Etiological Factor in Puerperal Breakdown 157

telling her mother of her engagement and of her first pregnancy. Her unconscious reason for this was that she had feared her mother's envy of her feminine successes and it seemed likely that her breakdown during pregnancy, resulting in the surrender of her baby to her mother, had occurred for similar reasons. She had not only to conceal her femininity from her real mother but, by extension, from all women and feared that people would think she had conceived her children too closely together.

Mrs. D. looked after her second baby lovingly, and took her other child, who was now mentally retarded, out of the residential nursery and began to look after her as well. After ten months in hospital she decided that she could now carry on successfully at home, which in fact she did.

Dread of Envy of Childbirth as a Feminine Achievement

The classical psychoanalytic view that childbirth is equated in the woman's mind with castration[2] does injustice to the positive aspects of this climax of feminine biological achievement. This view, based on Freud's theory that the feminine sexual drive is secondary to her primary penis-envy, has been criticised by Horney[3] and several other psychoanalysts. This is not to say that feelings of castration and loss do not have a place in the mind of many parturient mothers, especially those with a marked masculine identification (this will be discussed in the next section), but that such feelings have received exclusive attention in the past and consequently the success of childbirth, which may itself be envied, has not been given much thought.

That a puerperal mother will both fear envy and be envied is a logical consequence of Melanie Klein's belief that one of a child's most important feelings is envy of his mother's creative capacity.[4] Langer,[5] who bases her theoretical conclusions on the work of Melanie Klein, has studied a series of women who suffered from sterility or abortion, and concluded that an important etiological factor was the woman's fear of an envious (introjected) mother-figure.

The series of cases discussed in this chapter shows that this finding of Langer's also holds good in the sphere of puerperal breakdown. The dreaded envious mother-imago was sometimes projected on to a witchlike figure in the patient's environment. One mother was reluctant to return home because she had become terrified of a queer old woman who lived like a hermit in a neighbouring house. Witches are characteristically old, childless, ugly and deprived, envious of lucky young mothers, cause sterility and miscarriages, and take an especial delight in stealing and eating newborn children; and, as Ernest Jones[6] wrote 'Witches must be a personification of the hated and feared mother who is felt to be inimicable to the private wishes of the girl.'

That woman's creative capacity is envied not only by other women but also by men has been suggested both by psychoanalysts (especially Melanie Klein) and by anthropological studies[7]. It is likely, too, that feelings of envy contribute to the widespread practice of 'pseudo-maternal couvade' (Frazer),[8] in addition to the reasons which Reik,[9] has put forward to account for this phenomenon. Several of the patients in our series did fear the envy of men (one schizophrenic mother became convinced that her ex-husband would come back and steal her baby) but there was evidence that such a fear was often dependent on the masculine significance of childbirth, and this will now be considered.

Dread of Envy of Childbirth as a Masculine Achievement

Two cases, in which childbirth was felt by the mother to be primarily a masculine gain, will now be briefly described.

Case 5

Mrs. P. whose case I will discuss in more detail in the next chapter, was a woman of thirty-one, who had been admitted to a mental hospital where she was treated by electroconvulsive therapy, a few weeks after the birth of her third child, a boy. Her condition did not improve and she was admitted to hospital suffering from acute anxiety and an inability to stay at home and look after her baby who was by then 4 months old. For months she had a recurrent dream based on an episode she had witnessed at the mental hospital. The dream, in her own words, was as follows: 'There was a nice girl there with a young baby who had ECT and it did her no good. She was a very timid girl. They told her she must have insulin and she was terrified. She struggled on the stairs with the Sister who said "Don't be silly, if you don't have this treatment you'll never be able to have your baby back".'

In her associations to this dream Mrs. P. went on to say that she herself was terrified of insulin injections, but that she felt that to get better she would have to go back to the mental hospital and suffer this treatment. She had earlier stressed how she *must* keep her baby whatever else happened. This recurrent dream suggests that she felt she had to submit to an ordeal in order to be allowed to keep her baby, and, further, that this ordeal represented submission to sadistic intercourse (the injection).

She was a woman whose aims in life were directed by an intense rivalry with men, a rivalry based on a lifelong hatred and envy of her younger brother. She had married a man who was sick and disfigured and whom she dominated completely, and her pregnancy came as a surprise because she had believed him to be 'too weak to be fertile.'

Her baby reminded her of her younger brother and she felt a similar ambivalence towards him. Consciously she regarded childbirth as a failure of masculinity but unconsciously she felt it to be a phallic achievement, and she was able to take secret delight in her little boy's lively virility, and feared that he would be envied. The masochistic surrender in order to keep her baby, as depicted in the dream, may have been necessary because she felt him to be a stolen phallic possession.

Case 6

Mrs. F. was a woman of thirty-five who had suffered from depression and had been treated for several years by a psychiatrist, whom she idealized. During that time, with constant encouragement by him, she had conceived and borne a girl successfully. Her second child, a boy, was conceived without the blessing of her psychiatrist, and she bore the child with suffering and feelings of neglect. She spent the pregnancy looking after her sick and masochistic mother and organized a state of affairs whereby her mother looked after her sister (who was also pregnant) instead of herself.

After the baby was born she developed delusions that she smelt, that she was possessed by the Devil, and had lost God. As a result she was admitted to a mental hospital. She subsequently came to the Cassel Hospital with her baby, but grossly neglected him and made no attempt to prevent her savage and obsessional husband, who himself wanted to be the mother, from claiming him and taking him home.

She suffered from extreme envy of males, and it is significant that it was when she had a male child that she broke down. It is likely that she could not tolerate the guilt involved in the possession of masculinity that the birth signified. Also she lacked the blessing of a good father-figure (the psychiatrist or God) but was possessed by the evil father-figure (the Devil). The whole process seemed illicit in her mind, and her feeling of guilt and fear of envy forced her to give up her 'stolen' child to her husband. (That she needed to placate women, too, is suggested by her self-sacrificing care of her own mother during pregnancy).

Although, as was suggested earlier, the equation of childbirth with castration has been overemphasized in the literature, it is clear that a woman who has a great envy of men and to whom the baby which grows within her symbolizes the penis she has longed for, will feel childbirth as a castration and a loss. Zilboorg, in his paper on puerperal schizophrenia,[10] described a series of such mothers, and several of our cases confirmed his findings. However, because he adhered to the theory of primary penis envy, Zilboorg did not satisfactorily explain why such a mother could not recathect the baby after he was born, and feel him to be, as some mothers do, a valuable phallic possession. The reason why this kind of mother cannot do so would seem to be, first, that she is so narcissistic as to be not readily able to cathect an external object, and secondly, that she fears that to declare ownership of a baby, which represents a valuable but stolen penis, would incur the wrath and envy of those whom she had deprived.

The Symbolic Meaning of the Baby

A mother who has a healthy capacity to love values her baby primarily for what he is and only secondarily for his symbolic meaning. On the other hand, a less secure mother is likely to be primarily concerned with his value as a symbol. It is usually a phallic, or other idealized and envied attribute of a parent, that is symbolized, and often it is felt to be stolen, for which retaliation is expected. Insofar as splitting has occurred—a process facilitated by the regressed state in puerperal breakdown—the parent-imago will be divided into an idealized and a stolen part, symbolized by the baby and a deprived, envious, and retaliatory part either internal or projected (e.g., on to the witch or, as in the case of Mrs. F., the Devil).

To the extent that these idealized qualities possessed by the baby are accepted as part of the self, the baby will represent the mother as she has always wished to be. These qualities are not necessarily only idealized and unrealistic, but can be based on the projection of primitive wishes which have been pathologically repressed. This can be put another way by saying that the baby represents the 'real self,' as conceptualised by Winnicott.[11] This spontaneous behaviour, as it manifested itself in the patient as a child before it was defended against, or as it now manifests itself in her baby, is also liable to be felt by the patient as possibly stimulating envy in her own parents especially if (as in our series) they appear to be inhibited and embittered.

Masochistic Surrender to Ward Off Envy

Moral masochism was a prominent mechanism in the personality structure of the mothers studied, and it appeared that the problems brought to them by childbirth required the intense activation of this mechanism and seriously tested its stability. Dread of envy was one such problem for which a solution was attempted in this way. Insofar as this manoeuvre can be successful, the mother will behave masochistically at the time of childbirth, but will not suffer from a recognizable psychiatric illness. Where it fails she will suffer from acute anxiety (which will include a dread of envy) and will hastily erect defences against this. Many cases—and this includes most in our series—will exhibit masochistic behaviour as well as other symptoms. (It would, however, be an overstatement to say that excessive masochism during the puerperium is entirely a consequence of dread of envy, for feelings of guilt also contribute to this effect. If the mother feels that the quality envied is a real and genuine possession then her dread of envy will be simple; if, however, she feels it to be an alien quality which she has greedily stolen, then her dread of envy will be mixed with feelings of guilt. One would expect from this that it is likely to be the mother with a marked masculine identification who most suffers from guilt feelings and the cases quoted in this chapter suggest that this is so).

The mothers of this series needed to placate their parental introjects (and by extension the world in general) and this they did, sacrificing themselves by a public demonstration of maternal failure and suffering; sacrificing their babies through surrendering them to others; rejecting them and being unable to make contact with them or to love them; or even denying awareness of their existence. Looked at from this viewpoint, puerperal breakdown can be seen as a kind of ritual propitiation. Later (chapter 14) I shall discuss the extent to which behaviour similar to that described, occurring for similar reasons, can be observed in 'normal' mothers during the puerperium. There are many things which suggest that similar processes may occur; the taboo on the parturient mother in primitive society, the 'Churching of Women' in more modern times, and possibly, the degree of physical pain of childbirth. Remarkable, too, is the meekness of the woman in the maternity hospital, who will submit to all manner of deprivations without complaint, and with apparent willingness will let her function of feeding be usurped by that of the bottle, and—greatest deprivation of all—will permit separation from her baby and his removal to another room.

Conclusions

Dread of envy by others of the real or imagined attributes of a mother and her baby is one of the factors which threatens the mother's mental stability during the puerperium. It does so in at least three different ways:

1. This dread, acting directly, may reduce her to a state of acute anxiety and regression;
2. Because it is mainly directed towards her mother, or a substitute for her mother, it deprives her of an essential support at a crucial time;
3. A masochistic defence against this dread of envy may itself be sufficiently powerful to destroy her maternal capacity and even to reduce her to a state of psychiatric illness.

Acknowledgments

I wish to thank Dr. T. F. Main for his help and encouragement with this work and both Dr. Main and Dr. J. Davie for supplying me with some of the clinical material.

References

1. Deutsch, H. (1945), *Psychology of Women, vol. 2: Motherhood*, Research Books, London.
2. Abraham, K. (1927), 'Manifestations of the female castration complex,' in *Selected Papers*, Hogarth, London; Freud, S. (1948), 'The Economic Problem in Masochism,' in *Collected Papers, 2*, Hogarth, London.; Zilboorg, G. (1931), 'Depressive Reactions to Parenthood,' *Amer. J. Psychiat.* 10, p. 927; Deutsch, H., (1945), *Psychology of Women*.

3. Horney, K. (1948), 'On the genesis of the castration complex in women,' *Int. J. Psychoanal.* 5, p. 50.
4. Klein, M. (1957), *Envy and Gratitude: A Study of Unconscious Sources*, London, Tavistock.
5. Langer, M. (1958), 'Sterility and Envy,' *Int. J. Psychoanal.* 39, p. 129.
6. Jones, E. (1931), *On the Nightmare,* Hogarth, London and (1927) 'The Early Development of Female Sexuality,' *Int. J. Psychoanal.* 8, p. 459.
7. Mead, M. (1946), *Male and Female*, Gollancz, London; Bettleheim, B. (1956) *Symbolic Wounds*, Thames & Hudson, London.
8. Frazer, J. C. (1915), *The Golden Bough*, 3d ed., MacMillan, London.
9. Reik, T. ([1919] 1931), 'Couvade and the Psychogenesis of the Fear of Retaliation,' in *Ritual*, Hogarth, London.
10. Zilboorg, G. (1929),'The Dynamics of Schizophrenic Reaction to Pregnancy and Childbirth,' *Amer. J. Psychiat.* 8, p. 733.
11. Winnicott, D. W. (1958), 'Metapsychological and Clinical Aspects of Regression,' in *Collected Papers*, Tavistock, London.

11

The Husband-Wife Relationship in Cases of Puerperal Breakdown

Puerperal breakdown and the problems of maternity have been discussed by psychoanalysts almost entirely as phenomena dependent on the intrapsychic conflict present in the mother as a result of her faulty emotional development. This has resulted in neglect of the interpersonal relationships in the present which have a bearing on her illness. In this chapter a particular type of husband-wife relationship, which was found to exist to a varying degree in a series of cases of puerperal breakdown at the Cassel Hospital, and which seemed to have etiological significance, will be discussed.

One limitation of these observations is that they are based mainly on knowledge obtained from the mothers only, for it was the mothers who were treated; their husbands came directly into the therapeutic situation but rarely, although they were encouraged to visit the hospital as much as they liked and to sleep in at weekends. The series consisted of about a dozen mothers treated by the author over a period of two years, as well as a number of similar cases treated by hospital colleagues over the same period of time. This chapter describes impressions of dominant features in the husband-wife relationship in these cases, and which appear to have a specific relationship to puerperal breakdown. The mothers' problems have been described here in

---

Published in the *British Journal of Medical Psychology*, vol. 32, part 2, 1959, pp. 117–123.

terms of interpersonal relations. Intrapsychic factors, although of prime importance, have been rather left aside for the purposes of this exposition.

Husband-Wife Relationship prior to Breakdown

The total family constellation of these cases was similar to that described by Elizabeth Bott[1] as 'loose-knit'; that is to say that the links—(geographic, economic, and emotional) between present generation and past generation were weak, and the 'family' now consisted of husband, wife, and baby, and formed a relatively independent unit. In keeping with Bott's predictions there was no well-defined differentiation of roles between husband and wife. Within such a family structure deviations from a conventional masculine-feminine relationship are more likely to appear.

The most obvious deviation to be seen was a lack of femininity on the part of the wife to the extent usually of sexual frigidity; this was replaced by a dominating attitude towards her husband who assumed a passive role. This domination contained elements that could be described as sadistic, phallic, and maternal, in varying proportions from case to case. In several instances the domination was masked by an overtly masochistic attitude, but the husband remained the controlled partner just the same.

The concept 'maternal' is not a well-defined one, but if, following Winnicott[2] it is taken to mean an attitude of devotional care, characterized by empathy and requiring maturity, then these patients cannot be said to have possessed it to any significant degree. Their capacity to dominate and care for their husbands in a way that contained such phallic and sadomasochistic elements could perhaps best be called pseudo-maternal.

Mrs A. was a self-righteous woman with a deeply religious turn of mind and a distaste for sexuality, who felt herself to be living on a spiritual plane well above that of her husband, of whom she spoke with enormous contempt. He came from a class socially inferior to her own, and suffered from a recurring cerebral tumour; he was well enough to hold a job down but she spoke of him as being irresponsible to the point of imbecility.

Mrs D. was an ambitious career-girl who had always tried to rival men at their own game. She was almost totally frigid but spoke of her marriage as having been satisfactory in the past. She thought her husband unambitious and effeminate—a withdrawn man who pottered about the garden, did what he was told, and submitted meekly to her nagging. He wrote the therapist a gentle and humble letter in which his own wishes were not in evidence.

Mrs L. was one of the few mothers in the series who had a history of psychiatric illness prior to childbirth. She had been a midwife who had resorted to drugs in times of anxiety about her responsibilities at work. She was a quiet, withdrawn, masochistic woman, who felt herself to be deprived, and who, according to the psychologist's report 'can maintain quite good relationships with people who she can feel deprived like herself and to whom she can be of use.' The man she married was of the type one would expect of her: a quiet, lonely man who 'was not like most men who meet in pubs or take an interest in sport,' and who himself had had a nervous breakdown.

The impression gained from this series was that it was not only in the wife's fantasies that the husband was ineffectual and needy, but that her wish for such a mate had influenced her choice of selection in reality. A surprisingly high proportion of the husbands were physically sick men, and several of the wives had been professional nurses.

In spite of its pathological qualities this type of liaison was stable up to the time of childbirth, presumably because both parties were receiving considerable gratification from it. Insofar as the wife was concerned, this gratification could be explained not only by the sadomasochistic elements but by the narcissistic satisfaction involved.

According to Winnicott[3] the predominant fantasy in narcissistic states is that of the self being cared for by the mother with whom there is identification. These women could indulge in the fantasy of being the phallic mother who looked after the genitally deprived husband/child with whom she was also identified. As the hostility present was bound by the sadomasochistic element the relationship remained a closed system. It was ultimately unsatisfactory, however, for nearly all these patients desired real babies.

Owing to the fact that the husband's personality was not actually studied at first hand, his contribution to this set-up will not be discussed here; it is, however, important to note his passivity and dependence on his wife.

Reasons for Breakdown

The introduction of a baby into this system had disastrous results, and it is necessary to consider why an adjustment to the baby could not be made. Many factors, qualitative and quantative will decide the result in any particular case, but there would in general seem to be several possible outcomes to such a situation:

1. The wife could transfer her dominatingly maternal attitude onto the baby and leave the husband to his own resources.
2. The wife could adopt a maternal attitude to both husband and baby.
3. A change could occur in the family configuration in which the wife gained real satisfaction from real motherhood and the husband adopted a supporting role.
4. Puerperal breakdown could occur.

To take these in order:

1. In her paper 'Motherhood and sexuality,' Helene Deutsch[4] describes women, whom she calls, 'professional mothers,' who have successfully pursued this course. In her view, although difficulties of sexuality and of motherhood usually go hand in hand, the frigid woman often being sterile, there is frequently a split of varying intensity between sexuality and motherhood. She accounts for this split by saying that it is based on the denial of the loved mother as a person who would be so unfaithful as to have a sexual relationship with the father. The methods such women may adopt to maintain this split are described by her as:

a. flight into homosexuality;
b. the gaining of such masochistic satisfaction from motherhood that sexuality is unimportant;
c. variations of the parthenogenetic fantasy.

The last of these two mechanisms are relevant here. They are both based on a narcissistic fantasy similar to the one discussed, but the fantasy involves a real child and emphasis is laid on exclusion of the male. Deutsch describes women who adopt motherhood as a career to the exclusion of all else. The mothers in this series could very well have pursued the same path; they were keen to avoid sexuality, they gratified themselves masochistically to compensate for this, and some of them had parthenogenetic fantasies. (Mrs A., for instance, obsessionally perused gynecological textbooks in the hope of finding that the sperm made no contribution to the growth of the ovum), and they were keen to have many babies, being little discouraged even by their puerperal illness.

It is difficult to understand at first sight why they did not, in fact, become 'career' mothers, but several factors acted against this. Some of these will be discussed later, for they concern the reasons why these patients did in fact break down; they centre on the severity of maternal deficiency due to the intensity of sadomasochism. Another factor, present in some of these families, was that the intense emotional relationship and close identificatory bond between husband and wife would have made the independent pursuit of 'careers' difficult to achieve. The contemporary culture pattern may also play a part in that the belief that children should be allowed freedom of expression has made more difficult the position of the masochistic 'professional' mother, who possessively dominates her children without compunction; these mothers were very alive to this particular responsibility towards their babies, a responsibility which they found very troublesome.

2. The outcome of a maternal attitude to both husband and baby is unlikely, for the reason that there are practical and emotional limits to a woman's capacity to care for others if based on masochism, and this limit is likely to be reached during the puerperium more than at any time in her life.

3. A change in the family configuration with a favourable outcome would be possible if both husband and wife received such gratification and stimulation from parenthood that sadomasochism was lessened and they became capable of greater maturity.

4. Puerperal breakdown is, of course, this result with which we are concerned. The particular problems that would put a strain on a family such as has been described would be:
a. The mother is likely to find it difficult to adjust to the demands of a real baby owing to her deficiency in real maternal feeling, and the phallic and sadomasochistic elements in her personality. In the case of a mother who has a marked phallic attitude it can readily be understood that this would cause her to have serious difficulties with her

baby; and this could in fact be seen in some of the patients of this series. In the case of the masochistic mother, however, this is not so obvious as there is a widely held view that maternal love is in its very nature masochistic.

Helene Deutsch[5] has stressed the masochistic nature of motherhood, a view which is in keeping with her concept of 'essential feminine masochism.' There are, however, some reasons for doubting the value of this concept, which is based on the theory that female sexual desire is a secondary phenomenon. It seems likely then that what these patients lacked was real maternal love which is based not on a masochistic need to make reparation but a much more primary phenomenon. The whole question of the essential nature of mother love is, however, beyond the scope of this chapter. Nor will it be possible to discuss the diversity of problems which the sexual significance of childbirth and the identifications with the baby, whether boy or girl, will bring to the mother who has manifest severe sexual problems, although such factors were of great etiological significance in the cases of this series.

b. The mother, preoccupied with her baby and, for reasons outlined above, having greater emotional difficulties with him than even a 'normal' mother, has lost her capacity to support her husband and is now in urgent need of his support. The husband, in turn, finds new demands made on his self-reliance and on his own capacity to act as a source of strength to his wife, a role for which he has hardly received suitable training. It may be that some of the wife's scorn of her husband, which has been referred to, was on account of his actual failure to fulfil this role. Thus, at a time when her emotional life is disorganised, and she herself has lost her capacity to give support and is herself in desperate need of it, it is not forthcoming.

c. The introduction of a third party into a two-party system is always hazardous, but one would expect it to be particularly traumatic to a system that was based on narcissistic gratifications rather than on real object-relationships.

d. Owing to the loose-knit family organisation, with its social isolation and the unavailability of grandparents and other relatives, the mother was unable to draw on support other than that of her husband.

e. The problem brought by a changed cultural attitude towards the upbringing of children has already been mentioned. A family in which hostility is avoided by masochistic defences, and spontaneity is lacking, must have found the advent of a lively baby very difficult, especially if duty dictated a forbearing attitude towards the baby's excesses.

In the three cases described, the outcome was as follows:

Mrs A. developed a fear that she would kill her baby, became psychotically confused, and had to be admitted to an observation ward.

Husband-Wife Relationship in Cases of Puerperal Breakdown

After being discharged from there she would return neither to her husband nor to her baby, who was being cared for by her parents-in-law.

Mrs D. kept her baby, but left her husband and went to live with her mother. Her feelings for her baby were, however, anything but loving, and she felt him to be an unpleasant nuisance. When she came to the Cassel Hospital she practically disowned her husband, left the baby as far as possible to others, and expressed a determination never to return home.

Mrs L. did not openly express hostility to her husband or to the baby, but resorted to drug-taking to such a degree that threatened the baby's well-being, and was admitted to a mental hospital. The baby was placed in a residential nursery.

These examples were very typical of the series. Sometimes, as in the case of Mrs. D., the patient developed an open hate of her husband and baby; in other cases hate, which was originally concealed by symptoms such as anxiety, was revealed during the course of psychotherapy. A similar emotion of hate to husband and child on the part of the depressed puerperal mother was noted by Zilboorg.[6]

Many reasons could be found to account for the problem which the presence of the baby created for the mother, resulting in the anxiety and hate which she felt towards both husband and child, but one of the main reasons was that she simply could not tolerate the demands which in reality and in fantasy they made on her. She was tormented by the necessity to prove herself a good mother, and had obsessively to do her duty; this is one of the reasons why the masochistic woman is put under such a great strain by the arrival of a child.

That a nursing mother needs to be protected from the sexual demands of her husband is a fact well recognised in primitive society, which segregates husband and wife during the puerperium and establishes a taboo on sexual intercourse for a varying period, usually up to the time of weaning. These mothers, however, were troubled not only be the sexual needs of their husbands but by their husband's general dependence on them. 'I even have to manage the finances while I'm in hospital,' complained one mother.

These mothers could get their much-needed support neither from their husbands nor anyone else at home and so came to hospital for it. Thus, in addition to the intrapsychic conflict engendered in these patients by childbirth and the actual responsibility of a baby, they had to bear an additional burden imposed on them by the nature of their relationships with their husbands.

A more detailed description of one of the patients may help to illustrate some of these patterns.

Mrs P., a woman of thirty-one, has been chosen because her real family relationships were more overt than most, and because her symptoms demonstrate most clearly the pressure to which a mother could feel subjected by the changed family situation. In some ways, however, she was not typical of the series; although masochistic and often depressed, she had a more volatile personality than the other mothers, and her symptomatology included more hysterical features; she was the only mother to have been married before; and she proved to have the most intractable illness. In appearance Mrs. P. was a plump, vivacious, good-looking woman with a friendly yet somewhat challenging manner. She could remember remarkably little of her childhood, and practically nothing of her father, a waiter, who was regarded by her mother as a social inferior; nor did she remember her mother with any feeling of affection. She had a younger brother whom she now described, with a mixture of admiration and contempt, as a 'Cockney ruffian.' Her adult personality could be understood as having developed out of a need to escape from the family, to feel superior to it in terms of professional success and cultural achievement, and to compete with males.

Her first marriage, which took place when she was twenty, was a brief and unhappy wartime affair, supervised by her mother-in-law, and came to an end when her husband left her while she was in her second pregnancy. Although she felt devastated by her husband's desertion, she pulled herself together, and brought up two boys by her own efforts in spite of severe financial hardship. 'I was father and mother to them,' she said.

This independent, bisexual existence was not without enjoyment, but when the eldest boy was seven she sought a fresh husband. The man she chose was elderly, ailing, and disfigured, with a facial palsy and a discharging eye and ear—a pathetic figure who, on his own admission (later to the therapist) had never thought himself worthy of a woman's love. He was a foreman at the works where she was the boss's secretary, and she felt, as her own mother had, that she had married beneath her. Consciously she married him to gain financial security, but her choice was unconsciously directed by a need to have an abject partner to whom she could feel superior, and through whom she could gain her long awaited revenge on the male—represented in the past by the father who took little notice of her, the virile brother whom she envied, and the husband who deserted her.

The marriage worked satisfactorily for a while, but her triumph was brief, for to her utter surprise and dismay she conceived another child. Her contempt for her husband's virility had been so great that she had never believed he could be fertile and had not taken the necessary precautions to prevent conception. (One cannot help feeling that a need to punish herself for her revenge lay behind this foolhardy attitude, quite apart from an unconscious wish for another child).

After having the baby (a boy) she became filled with anxiety and was unable to remain at home, moving from house to house, sometimes with the baby or sometimes without, and was sent to a mental hospital where she was treated by electroconvulsive therapy without improvement. She was finally admitted to the Cassel Hospital with her baby, in a state of the most desperate anxiety. The picture she painted was akin to the nightmare of the *Sorcerer's Apprentice*: her husband, her two other children, the washing up, the nappies, and the baby's crying tormented her. She was tremendously impatient with the baby and felt he should immediately do whatever she wanted. The type of transference that she developed towards her (male) therapist was such as would be expected of a frigid woman with an envy of men—she showed the greatest contempt for the therapist's interpretations, forgetting them as soon as she was out of the room and became locked with him in an endless struggle for ascendency. It was this transference that made her so difficult to treat, and it is likely that a similar situation would have occurred in treatment at any period of her life.

What we are most concerned with here are the problems caused by the birth of the child. The important ones, revealed during the course of a year's treatment, can be briefly categorized as follows:

1. Problems caused by identification with the baby: these included punishment by the superego for the vicarious gratification of primitive desires, and a fear of greed and sadism which had been projected on to the baby;

2. Guilt arising from the unconscious masculine success involved in producing a boy;

3. A breakdown of a previously stable relation to her husband

from which she received the gratification of feeling masculine, superior, and maternally giving, and its replacement by a situation in which she finds herself feeling dependent on him (which hurts her pride), at the same time being unable to receive support from him. Thus the acute anxiety, which was her main symptom, and which at times reduced her to a state in which she screamed or talked hysterically and incoherently, seemed to be due to the fact that she felt herself surrounded by tremendous demands which she could not satisfy. Whereas before the childbirth she had been the family leader, she now could not bear her husband to leave her, and wept helplessly when her child dirtied the house. Her husband was in fact not capable of firmness and she herself had insufficient respect for him to find him a source of strength. Due to her sorry plight, and the sympathy she aroused in others, she was the only patient in the series to be readmitted. She returned, in a state of desperation, complete with baby and baggage and demanded to be allowed to come back. This could be seen as a combination of separation anxiety, of her desire to control, her fear of passivity, and a flight from her family to whose demands she had no answer. The distress of this woman was not only manipulative technique but was very real and pathetic; she was bitterly ashamed that she could not respond to the demands of motherhood.

In thinking about this mother, the question naturally comes to mind: why did she break down now and not when she had her first two babies? One can do no more than speculate, but there was one important difference in the two situations: her relationship with her first husband, as far as one could tell, was of quite a different nature from the typical one described in this chapter, for he was an aggressive and independent man who would neither tolerate her bossiness, nor make demands on her maternal capacity.

In this particular husband-wife set-up the phallic elements in the wife's personality and her sadistic and revengeful domination of her husband were very obvious. His contribution to her breakdown consisted in his inability (in reality) to act as a support to her and in his demand (in her fantasy) for reparation, as a result of her sadism against him and triumph over him.

In the cases in this series in which the patient's attitude to her husband, although dominating, contained more apparently positive and maternal elements, the mechanism of breakdown of husband-wife relationship seemed to be not essentially different from that outlined in this last case, but was less conscious. In these cases the sadistic elements in the relationship had been bound by masochism and idealism, the baby was openly desired, worries about childbirth was denied, and puerperal breakdown came as a terrible surprise and shock, bringing the mother to a state of acute anxiety.

Conclusion

In this chapter puerperal breakdown is considered from the viewpoint of the husband-wife relationship before and after breakdown. A particular type of relationship which has been observed to exist with some consistency, and which is thought to have etiological significance, is described and discussed.

Acknowledgements

I wish to express my thanks to Dr. T. F. Main for his help and encouragement with this work.

References

1. Bott, E. (1957), *Family and Social Network*, Tavistock, London.
2. Winnicott, D. ([1956] 1958), 'Primary Maternal Preoccupation,' in *Collected Papers*, Tavistock, London.
3. Winnincott, D. ([1954] 1958), 'Withdrawal and Regression,' in *Collected Papers*, Tavistock, London.
4. Deutsch, H. (1933), 'Motherhood and Sexuality,' in *Psychoanaly. Quart.* 2, p. 476.
5. Deutsch, H. (1947), *Psychology of Women, vol. 2: Motherhood*, Research Books, London.
6. Zilboorg, G. (1931), 'Depressive Reactions Related to Parenthood,' *Amer. J. Psychiat.* 10, pp. 927–962.

12

The Concept of Maternal Love

According to psychoanalytic theory, maternal love derives much of its strength from elements of narcissism and masochism in the mother's personality. This conception, which is in conflict with many observations of normal and abnormal mothering, will be explored in this chapter and an attempt made to show in what way it fails to explain the healthy mother's spontaneous love for her baby.

Freud, in a 1914 work, writes: 'If we look at the attitude of fond parents towards their children, we cannot but perceive it as a revival and reproduction of their own, long since abandoned narcissism. Their feeling, as is well known, is characterized by over-estimation, that sure indication of a narcissistic feature in object-choice which we have already appreciated ...'[1]

Helene Deutsch's conception of maternal love includes both narcissistic and masochistic elements. She writes:

> I have defined as characteristic of the feminine woman a harmonious interplay between narcissistic tendencies and masochistic readiness for painful giving and loving. In the motherly woman, the narcissistic wish to be loved, so typical of the feminine woman, is metamorphasized; it is transferred from the ego to the child or his substitute. However, it can be clearly observed that despite this altruistic transformation the narcissistic elements are preserved. For instance, the mother's love for the child is often associated with the fact that she considers herself absolutely and exclusively indispensable to him ... The masochistic components of

---

Reprinted from *Psychiatry, Journal for the Study of Interpersonal Processes*, 25, 3 (1962)

motherliness manifest themselves but in the mother's readiness for self-sacrifice, but ... without demand for any obvious return on the part of the object, ie. the child, and also her willingness to undergo pain for the sake of her child's dependence upon her when his hour of liberation comes.*

It is necessary to reconcile these views with the well-established knowledge that narcissistic or masochistic qualities in a mother can be harmful both to her child's psychology and to her own—that is, these qualities commonly interfere with maternal capacity, and predispose a mother to puerperal breakdown.[2]

A further reason for questioning the idea of the biological normality of maternal masochism is that it is based on the theory that the feminine sexual drive is secondary to her primary penis-envy, a theory that would be unacceptable to many psychoanalysts today.

The Relationship between Narcissism and Masochism

When used to denote certain kinds of pathological behaviour, the terms *narcissism* and *masochism* have relatively clear meanings. Their exact connotation, however, is uncertain and the subject of much debate among psychoanalysts, as is the question of how far such concepts can be usefully applied to normal, healthy phenomena.

One essential difference between narcissism and masochism would seem to be that whereas in the former it is the subject that overtly commands interest, in the latter it is the object. The narcissist indulges in self-gratification and self-idealization; the masochist gains pleasure from painful submission to an idealized object. This can be put in

---

*Since the formulations of Freud and Deutsch, relatively little has been written on this subject. Studies of the mother-child relationship have been preoccupied with the child's psychology, rather than the mother's, with the result that criticism of the classical psychoanalytical theory of maternal love has been mainly by implication only. See, for example: John Bowlby, 'The Nature of the Child's Tie to His Mother,' *Int. J. Psychoanal.* (1958) 39:350-373; Erik H. Erikson, *Childhood and Society* (New York, Norton, 1950); Rene A. Spitz, *No and Yes: On the Genesis of Human Communications* (New York, Internat. Univ. Press, 1957); and D. W. Winnicott, *Collected Papers: Through Paediatrics to Psycho-Analysis* (New York, Basic Books, 1958). Winnicott has at times focused his attention directly on the psychology of the mother (see, for example, 'Primary Maternal Preoccupation,' pp. 300-305, in *Collected Papers*); he has not, however, attempted to reassess classical theory on the basis of his findings.

terms of psychoanalytic theory by saying that in narcissism there is an excess of subject libido, and in masochism, of object libido.

The similarity between the two concepts is, however, more fundamental than the difference. For example, schizophrenic withdrawal—an extreme form of narcissism—involves a sacrificial social annihilation and compensatory passive gain. Similarly, the masochist, although apparently submitting to the object, is preoccupied with physical gratification, moral self-idealization, or concealed omnipotent control. Narcissism and masochism are similar in being defensive manoeuvres designed to avoid the impact of a full and spontaneous relationship with another person. By means of emphasis on one of the two participants rather than on their mutual relationship, by identificatory mechanisms, and by denial of hostility, a controlled experience occurs in which the unpredictable and frightening creative union of two real people is avoided.

The confusion of terminology appears to derive from the fact that people have a healthy capacity which at first sight seems similar to the pathological attitudes described, but is not only distinct from them but also diametrically opposed to them. This is the capacity to become so absorbed by and secure in a relationship that questions of the relative importance of self and object, of control and dependency, do not arise, with the consequence that a real, spontaneous delight in either self or object can be safely indulged in. This type of 'narcissism' is not accompanied by guilt or precarious pride for it does not involve any comparison with the object, and such a 'masochist' can worship and surrender to the object without any self-degradation. It is doubtful whether there is any value in retaining these terms in this usage.

The Economy of the Mother-Child Relationship

The conception of the mother-child relationship as a masochistic-narcissistic one is influenced by the traditional view that in a relationship of unequal degrees of autonomy libido flows from one to the other; the child gains by taking from the mother, who willingly accepts this loss to herself because of her innate masochism; any gain the mother might herself receive is not derived from simple interaction with the child but is narcissistic and based on illusion. In a paper in which he discusses the use of the concept of entropy in the economy of human relationships Szasz challenges this view:

> ... *in order for one person to benefit (grow), the interaction must be beneficial for both.* If it is not, the hidden damage to the recipient person (be this the child, the recipient of charity, the analytic patient, etc) in the form of feelings of guilt, responsibility, or a much vaguer feeling of 'being weighed down' with the suffering of the giver may be so great as to outweigh the gain in care, information, or maturation coincident with the association between the participants. It must be remembered that in all the foregoing interpersonal phenomena the nature of the human contact is such that each individual relates meaningfully to the other, as a like individual. By 'meaningful' we simply mean that A considers B (and vice versa) to be fundamentally 'human,' that is, more or less like himself. This definition of 'human relationship' would therefore encompass only a small proportion of all those social processes that actually occur in nature, as we now know it. [3]

This formulation, which calls to mind Buber's differentiation between *I-Thou* and *I-It* relationships, is entirely in accord[4] with the view of maternal love taken in this chapter.*

Although a sacrificial withdrawal from life may appear to characterize the devoted mother and justify the use of the term masochistic, the withdrawal is only apparent because the mother's milieu includes the baby. She does not withdraw from objects but concentrates on one particular object. She denies herself only in the sense that all concentration involves relinquishing of other interests. She does not sacrifice herself to the baby but becomes—to use Winnicott's term—'preoccupied' with him.[5]

The masochistic mother, however, is incapable of deriving the satisfaction and stability of a full emotional engagement with a baby and is dependent on the maintenance of certain precarious balances of forces which may get upset in various ways:

1. The self-assertion and exhibitionism that accompanies successful childbirth may prove incompatible with the demands of her strict superego.
2. Identification with the baby's uninhibited behaviour may also cause conflict with the superego.
3. The baby may not remain sufficiently happy to supply her with the vicarious gratification—by projective identification—on which she depends.
4. The overwhelming demands made by a lively baby may be intolerable and may overstrain the masochistic defenses against anger.

---

* This erroneous concept of love is not restricted to the field of theory. The reason why patients often regard a love experience as one in which they obtain some kind of nutriment from the other person has been discussed by Albert E. Scheflen in 'A Common Defect in Extrapolation: Explaining Psychic and Social Processes in Terms of Feeding,' *Psychiatry* (1961) 24, pp. 143–152.

5. Those around her may not appreciate her sacrificial care of the baby to the extent that she requires them to do so.

If there is an unfavourable imbalance of these forces, the mother will be unable to care for her child even superficially—and may herself fall victim to overt mental illness. A masochistic woman who regards herself as a virtuous and loving person and a potentially successful mother may experience immense shame over her maternal failure and may completely lose her belief in herself. What had previously passed for love is revealed as a facade of love. The only insurance against such an occurrence is the possession of real maternal love.

Love toward another human being—as opposed to that toward an inanimate object which can be brought under control—is characterised by flexibility. An artist or scientist may have a passionate interest in his work that is often called 'love of his work,' but love differs from this interest in relating to an object possessing an agency and spontaneity of its own which requires recognition of its uniqueness and unpredictability. Maternal love can be considered in several different ways:

1. The mother perceives her child as an individual, yet also as a member of a class, deviation from which may indicate ill health.
2. She perceives him as an individual whose autonomy needs respect, yet also as a possession inasmuch as she is ultimately responsible for him and at certain times must interfere with his autonomy.
3. She is sufficiently aware of her own primitive and dependent needs to have empathy with him, yet remains sufficiently detached from them to avoid the temptation of indulging in these needs herself.
4. She has an attitude of mature and detached concern for his needs although experiencing undetached and intense feelings of adoration and physical gratification.
5. She is able to combine the feminine quality of receptivity which enables her to 'hold' the baby,* with functions which can easily symbolise masculine activity. For example, breast-feeding sometimes has the unconscious symbolic meaning of a phallic activity.
6. Her love object, constantly changing, starts as a fetus and ends up a mature and independent adult.

Some of these points require further consideration.

---

*I am using the word *hold* not only in its narrow physical connotation but also in a more general sense which would include all those psychological activities by the mother that result in the child's feeling that he exists safely within a firm relationship. In doing this I am following Winnicott's usage of the term.

The Nature of the Love Impulse

Assertion of the spontaneity of maternal love involves a criticism of the psychoanalytic conception of love itself. However, in the context of this chapter, such criticism can only be made very briefly.

According to Freud, object-relationships are of two types, anaclitic, or narcissistic—that is, based on self-interest. The narcissistic type he regards as characteristic of women:

> Even for women whose attitude towards the man remains cool and narcissistic there is a way which leads to complete object-love. In the child to whom they give birth, a part of their own body comes to them as an object other than themselves, upon which they can lavish out of their narcissism complete object-love.[6]

However, the maternal object-love to which Freud refers retains the narcissistic qualities discussed above, and the child is attractive not of itself but only insofar as it represents the mother.

The theory that object-relations have their origin in narcissism has been criticised by several psychoanalysts, in particular, Balint, Klein, and Fairbairn.

Fairbairn writes:

> The ultimate goal of libido is the object, and in its search for the object libido is determined by similar laws to those which determine the flow of electrical energy, i.e., it seeks the path of least resistance. The erotogenic zone should, therefore, be regarded simply as a path of least resistance: and its actual erotogenicity may be likened to the magnetic field established by the flow of an electrical current.[7]

A similar kind of criticism has been made by writers outside the psychoanalytic school. Tillich writes:

> First of all it must be said that libido is misunderstood if it is defined as the desire for pleasure ... But it is not the pleasure as such which is desired, but the union with that which fulfils the desire. Certainly, fulfilled desire is pleasure, and unfulfilled desire is pain. But it is a distortion of the actual processes of life if one derives from these facts the pain-pleasure principle in the sense that life essentially consists in fleeing from pain and striving for pleasure. Whenever this happens life is corrupted.[8]

The 'corruption' of which Tillich writes would seem to be akin to what is described in psychoanalytic terminology as 'splitting.' The purity of a simple, direct, and complete relationship is destroyed by a process in which emphasis is laid on one aspect of the relationship at the expense of the whole. Another word which could well be used in this context is 'degradation,' which means not only a 'lowering of dignity' but a 'change from a higher to a lower level of complexity'—that is, a disintegration.

The overemphasis given by theory to the physical aspect of the love impulse has resulted from the difficulty of presenting a scientifically respectable account of love in an era in which conceptions are accounted valid only if based on physical evidence, and what is considered physical in relation to human beings is that which is left over when the 'mind' has been extracted. The fallacy lies in the false body-mind dichotomy which has, until recently, remained unchallenged as a philosophical truth. This conceptual error is an example of the parallel which often occurs between academic formulations and practical living, for patients become involved in a similar error when they salvage pleasure from a disintegrated love relationship by an overvaluation of certain elements of it, thus making a narcissistic or masochistic adaptation to life.

It may be urged that although the mature love impulse is not based on narcissism it is genetically preceded by it, in accordance with Freud's formulations. An attempt to combat this argument is not necessary in order to establish the concept of maternal love put forward here, and is therefore beyond the scope of this chapter, but it is worth mentioning that: (1) the above considerations hold good for infantile life also, and (2) serious criticisms of Freud's theory of infantile narcissism have been made on the basis of child observation. Schachtel maintains that: man's grasp of reality is not merely based on his wish to satisfy primary, biological needs—is not merely, as Freud assumed, a detour on the path of wish fulfilment—but that it also has as prerequisite an autonomous interest in the environment.[9]

Relieved from the necessity of deriving love from the theory of infantile narcissism, one can see that love grows out of a diffuse awareness of life, beginning as a simple and spontaneous delight in a relationship that is already in existence and an urge to maintain and increase that relationship to the fullest extent, using all possible modes of communication. As such it is a primary state of being, the occurrence of which is no more explicable than is being itself.

The Mother's Perception of Her Child

The loving mother's perception of her child has a different quality from that of the impartial observer. To her he is 'Johnny'; to the observer he is a 'child' or a 'boy,' a member of a class, albeit, perhaps, with particular characteristics. These two types of perception are fundamentally different, but, as the existential school has shown, each have a claim to the term 'realistic.' The former type views the other person in his uniqueness and immediacy, does not set him at a distance in order to analyze, is unfettered by rigid preconceptions, and, because it occurs within a relationship, observes the other in spontaneous action, a perception denied to all observers who do not fully engage him.

From the pragmatic point of view, also, there is reason to suppose that the healthy mother's perception of her child's individuality is realistic. Studies of the families of schizophrenics—for example, those of Wynne and co-workers[10]—show that the lack of development of a sense of identity, characteristic of this illness, occurs in children whose families perceive them not as individuals but as rigid units in a system. This finding suggests that a necessary feature of a healthy parental attitude is an accurate perception of the child's particularity and that a parent who lacks this type of perception is being dangerously unrealistic.

It seems probable, however, that it is the individualised type of perception by the mother that has led to the belief that her attitude toward her child is unrealistic, for should she wish to convey her unique experience of her child to others she cannot do so in ordinary language. In this respect she is in the position of the artist but without his special ability to create new symbolic forms of communication. In trying to express her experience of her baby's supreme significance and uniqueness she will fall prey to the use of logically untenable superlatives and comparisons and will risk being thought of as indulging in narcissistic overestimation.

This type of perception is perhaps maximal during the state of 'primary maternal preoccupation' that lasts for a few weeks after childbirth and is characterised by heightened sensitivity, difficult to communicate.

In addition to the charge of narcissistic overvaluation, the type of maternal perception described here might well be open to the general criticism of resembling that of the infant both in its association with strong emotion and its lack of logical analysis. The theory that emotion is inimicable to the pursuit of the truth is debatable, and from a biological point of view it is to be expected that an organism operating to its full capacity, and therefore experiencing life to the full, would also be functioning adequately intellectually. Certainly a frustrated wish can lead away from reality to the primary-process mechanism of hallucinatory wish-fulfilment, but it may equally lead to the pursuit of what is wished for and to an intellectual concentration on the realities which will enable that goal to be reached. It is not because of his urges that an infant's perception of the world is limited.

Another clue to the character of maternal perception can be found in a second characteristic of infantile perception, the lack of differentiation. This characteristic does limit his realistic view of the world, but this negative description leads one to overlook its positive aspect—namely, the capacity to see the whole in a direct and simple manner that is denied under the more sophisticated and abstract functioning of logical analysis. It is this function that is the origin of the type of maternal perception discussed above, which sees the child as a real, unique, and human being. Such perception involves the infant—and the mother—in a particular type of belief, the belief of fusion and essential belongingness, which Alice Balint noted and regarded as a sign of the mother's lack of realism.[11] Classical psychoanalytic theory similarly regards such a belief on the part of the baby to be unrealistic. Even Milner, who has shown its importance in child development and creative achievement, refers to it as 'illusion.'[12] But just as scientific analysis has concealed the truth of the uniqueness of persons, so it may conceal their essential inseparability.*

It would therefore seem that although elements of maternal love involve a type of perception typically infantile, these characteristics do not of themselves constitute distortions of reality. If the mother's love were to show itself identical with infantile love it would undoubtedly be deemed unrealistic, for her child would be hopelessly neglected and would die. Fortunately maternal love also shows the characteristics of mature (genital) love, as defined by Balint. 'In order to win a loving

---

*The fusion of self and object in primitive thought, usually regarded as a distortion of reality under the influence of wish, could be the infant's symbolic expression in concrete imagery of this essential unity. Moreover, a theory of wish-fulfilment which assumes that the infant's overriding need is for fusion overlooks the possibility that the infant may have an equal need for differentiation, a need to discover and have confirmed the confines of what Winnicott terms his 'real self' (see Winnicott, note 2).

and lovable genital object and to keep it for good,' he writes, 'nothing can be taken for granted as happens in oral love; a permanent, never-relaxing, exacting reality testing must be kept up all the time.'[13]

The drive toward this attitude develops during growth partly as a result of a greater appreciation of the various needs of the object and partly because of conformity to a moral code which demands such an attitude. It can be achieved because of the increased capacity to stand aside from the full experience of the relationship as it is actually occurring in order to conceptualize and therefore make necessary changes. This involves a sacrifice of immediate experience, but a gain in long-term result and in the sheer delight of conceptual thinking and technical ability; it cannot be called masochistic without stretching the use of that term to include all mature behaviour.

The Difficulty of Conceptualizing Maternal Love

It is less easy to say what maternal love is than what it is not. Past formulations have erred by including elements which are neither essential nor healthy, although they exist in mothers in Western culture. Similar errors occur in attempts to define, say, masculinity or femininity, because the observer is not neutral and tends to regard the average of his culture as the natural, essential, and desirable. Moreover, the conceptions which the observer brings to the question are couched in the terms of his philosophical outlook. It was probably as difficult to write a treatise on maternal love in medieval times without basing it on the notion of Divine Love as it is today without centering on a particular theory of biological drive. One of the difficulties also seems to lie in the observer's distance from the actual experience. The people who could best tell whether maternal love is in operation and what it is like are the mother and child, provided they were able and prepared to communicate this. But they are most likely to communicate it not by a conception but by demonstrating happiness, health, and growth. When maternal love fails it becomes easier to formulate what is going on.

Perhaps I might summarize my position by saying that maternal love is based neither on defense mechanisms nor compromise adaptations such as narcissism and masochism, but is a full engagement of the baby, based, as is love in general, on a primary, spontaneous, and realistic interest in the outer world.

References

1. Freud, Sigmund (1914), 'On Narcissism,' in *Collected Papers*, 4, Hogarth, London, p. 48.
2. Deutsch, Helene (1945) *The Psychology of Women, vol. 2: Motherhood*, Grane & Stratton, p. 15.
3. Szasz, Thomas S. (1955), 'Entropy, Organization and the Problem of the Economy of Human Relationships,' *Int. J. Psychoanal* 36, p. 291.
4. Buber, Martin (1937), *I and Thou*, translated by R. Gregor Smith, T. Edinburgh, and T. Clarke.
5. Winnicott, D.W. (1958), 'Primary Maternal Preoccupation,' in *Collected Papers*, Basic Books, New York.
6. Freud, Sigmund, 'On Narcissism.'
7. Fairbairn, W. R. D. (1952), *Psychoanalytic Studies of the Personality*, Tavistock, London, p. 31.
8. Tillich, Paul (1954), *Love, Power and Justice*, Oxford University Press, London, p. 28.
9. Schachtel, Ernest G. (1954), 'The Development of Focal Attention and the Emergence of Reality,' *Psychiatry* 17, p. 309
10. Wynne, L. C., I. M. Ryckoff, J. Day, and S. I. Hirsch (1958), 'Pseudo-Mutuality in the Family Relations of Schizophrenics,' *Psychiatry* 21, pp. 205–220.
11. Balint, Alice (1952), 'Love for the Mother and Mother Love,' pp. 109–127, in *Primary Love and Psychoanalytic Technique*, by Michael Balint, Hogarth, London.
12. Milner, Marion (1957), *On Not Being Able to Paint*, International Universities Press, New York.
13. Balint, M. (1952), *Primary Love and Psychoanalytic Technique*, Hogarth, London, p. 135.

13

An Interpretation of Modern Obstetric Practice

Let me be open at the start and say that I am among those who have serious doubts about the rationale of modern obstetric practice. I have been led to this position through my work as a psychotherapist, and in particular by my attempts to help mothers suffering from post-partum depression. But, although my views on the subject will emerge in what follows, I am, in this chapter, primarily concerned with understanding the phenomenon rather than writing a polemic about it.

If we view childbirth from the psychological point of view, and are concerned with the immediate or long-term effects of the way the mother and baby, considered as persons, are treated by society, then we may query the legitimacy of the current preoccupation with techniques, may challenge their presumed necessity, and, to the extent that we doubt their wisdom, may try to understand why behaviour which we consider inappropriate should become widely accepted.

As a first approach one must, I feel, draw a distinction between those elements which pervade our society and colour attitudes not only to childbirth but to many areas of living, and, on the other hand, elements that are specific to childbirth itself (while recognizing, of course, that the two cannot be entirely separated). It is clear that,

---

Published in *The Place of Birth,* ed. Kitzinger, S. and Davis, J. Oxford University Press (1978) This was a revised edition of 'Ritualistic Elements in the Management of Childbirth,' *British Journal of Medical Psychology,* 39, p. 207 (1967).

amongst the former, the phenomenon of current medical practice is of paramount importance. Childbirth may be subjected to various dominating influences. It could, for instance, be the occasion of a religious ceremony or festival, in which the midwife assumed a secondary role. But in our society childbirth is first and foremost a medical matter. The doctor and the gynecologist are the authorities who, in the main, prescribe the circumstances of the birth, which takes place in their buildings and under their guidance and control.

Civilisation is the process of taming the wild, because the wild is hazardous and terrifying. We cannot eliminate the terror of living but we can make some areas more secure than they were for earlier man. Medicine, based on contemporary scientific principles, helps to preserve life and reduce disease. If it were as simple as that, a critique of obstetric practice could be straightforward. But, for various reasons (including the following), we cannot take the beneficial influence of medicine for granted.

First, medicine can bring harmful side-effects and illness.

Secondly, despite the medical profession's doctrine of belief that medicine is about the whole person, and even though doctors, nurses, and midwives are human beings (rather than mere agents of a scientific viewpoint), who will, by and large, treat their patients as human beings, medicine tends to neglect the whole person.

Thirdly, there is the effect of monopoly. As with other branches of science, the success of and belief in medical technology ensures ever-expanding boundaries even in the face of its notable failures. We no longer go to the doctor only when we are sick, we consult him in health; and the pregnant woman puts herself under his care. But we have to ask the question: 'Is there a threshold beyond which the influence of medical science is counterproductive?' And to take note of Illich's suggestion that our capacity to look after ourselves is threatened by the tendency to rely on experts.[1]

Fourthly, medicine is increasingly controlled by a uniform, centralized policy, with an inevitable increase in impersonality. The relevant question here is 'Can such a personal experience as childbirth be adequately managed in a setting that is orientated towards the impersonal?'

Before pursuing the argument further, I would like to present a brief description of the modern obstetric practice. In what follows I shall outline a pattern of social behaviour which, although by no means

An Interpretation of Modern Obstetric Practice

universal, has significance, in most of its elements, for a large number of mothers in the technological society of the mid-twentieth century. As such it represents an oversimplified model and the fact that it has probably by now passed its peak does not invalidate an attempt to understand the phenomenon.

The Modern Obstetric Regime

1. During pregnancy the mother is advised about conduct beneficial or harmful to the baby, laying emphasis on foodstuffs. She may be warned against having sexual intercourse.
2. In many, if not most, cases, arrangements are made for her to be confined away from her home and family. If this does occur the family is excluded from the procedure and its contact with the mother is strictly limited.
3. The birth is medically induced, i.e., the timing is not left to natural physiological processes but is controlled by means of drugs.
4. The mother is confined to bed during the whole process.
5. The birth area is shaved.
6. Drugs are given to relieve pain and to stimulate labour.
7. The mother is moved from the room in which she has been labouring to a different room in the hospital in order to give birth.
8. For the birth to take place the mother is laid flat on her back, with her knees drawn up and spread wide apart by stirrups.
9. Childbirth is expected to be a painful process. The mother characteristically moans or screams, and in general behaves in a rather helpless way, and is spoken to as though she were a child (and often a naughty child).
10. In many cases the birth takes place under anaesthesia.
11. Pressure is sometimes applied to the abdomen during delivery.
12. In some areas the baby is delivered by instruments as a normal, routine measure.
13. A surgical incision is made the enlarge the vaginal orifice.
14. The umbilical cord is clamped immediately after birth.
15. The expulsion of the placenta is hastened by pulling the cord, pressing the abdomen, and the use of drugs.
16. After the birth and for the length of her stay in hospital the mother is separated from her baby for at least part of the time in many hospitals. He is looked after by the staff, in a room together with other babies, and presented to the mother only for brief periods, primarily for the purpose of feeding.
17. The baby is sometimes weighed before being handed to the mother.
18. Feeding of the baby is delayed. Later he is given modified cow's milk taken from a bottle at scheduled times.

Setting aside the question of the medical usefulness of these measures (a question which will be confronted elsewhere in this book) we can ask 'Is there a pattern or trend in these practices which can help us to understand why they should be performed? Looked at naively, what is happening to mother and baby?' Certain (interrelated) elements quickly reveal themselves:

a. Both mother and baby are placed in a very passive position. The mother's contribution to the birth is almost the minimal conceivable; the process is taken out of her hands and her body is manipulated by professionals. The professionals come as near to having the baby themselves as can be managed by proxy. And afterwards even her baby is removed from her.
b. The occasion is one of suffering rather than of joy.
c. The impersonal mode is ascendant; spontaneity is replaced by control; the significance of psychological reality is denied.
d. There is a break of continuity in the mother's life; the birth does not take place in her ordinary place of living.
e. Great emphasis is put on cleanliness (purity) and order.
f. There is a formality which has something of the character of public ritual.

These are the trends that I wish to underline. Even after as much credence as possible has been given to medical justification for this practice, and even when allowance has been made for the effects of rationalistic-technological philosophy, the phenomenon is sufficiently striking to make us wonder about the meanings that may lie behind it. At a period of history when the importance of individual rights and freedom of expression is not in doubt, how can an obstetric regime so antipathetic to these rights gain wide acceptance? When the significance of the early mother-baby tie and of the need to allow basic bodily and emotional drives their due consideration is recognized, not only be psychiatry but by a large proportion of the educated public, how can the potential harm of intrusive control be overlooked? Why do professional helpers so usurp the mother's function and why does she let this happen? These are questions I hope to leave in the reader's mind. In what follows I shall make an attempt to shed some light on them and in particular, to explore possible reasons for the existence of a cultural attitude to childbirth that is far less positive than we would like to believe.

The meaning of a pattern of social behaviour is always more extensive than the explanation given by the participants; indeed, the anthropologist's work rests on this assumption. But, as Cohen suggests, research into underlying meanings are too often reserved for the study of 'primitive society.'[2]

The view, implicit in the evolutionary formulations of Weber and others, that modern society is distinct from primitive society in being organised on the basis of contract, in being secular, rational, manipulative, and impersonal, has recently been seriously challenged by many students of society. A rapidly accumulating body of evidence indicates that the bizarre and the exotic in the patterns of social behaviour are not the exclusive monopoly of pre-industrial societies. In many situations in modern society, custom is as strange and as sovereign as it is in 'primitive' society.

Scholars are now 'rediscovering' in modern society the existence and significance of an endless array of patterns of symbolic behaviour that have been for long associated exclusively with 'primitive' society.

What might these hidden patterns be in relation to obstetric method? We do not regard the practices surrounding childbirth in our society as ceremonial or ritualistic, but may the ritual be hidden from us only because we are so hypnotised by the apparently rational assumptions behind them that we do not even begin to seek a further explanation? Such overt ceremonials as we have available to us—Christian baptism and churching of women—are gradually paling into insignificance in the face of the powers of the doctor and the hospital. It is well known that when a social order is superseded, the old customs are not thereby automatically extinguished but will persist in modified forms. For instance, several elements of the Mithraic religion have found their way into Christian ceremony and theology, and much of the spirit of the Jewish sabbath has continued to pervade the Christian Sunday. May this kind of thing happen when the priest is replaced by the doctor, and the church by the hospital? If this is so, then hospitals may be places where propitiation and blessing play a greater part than we imagine.*

---

* Cf. L.R. Twentyman in 'The place of homeopathy in modern medicine in the light of history': 'It would be very superficial also to ignore or underestimate the symbolic elements in modern medicine and surgery and their influence for good and ill in activating unconscious forces. The ritual of the modern operating theatre is an example. There is the sacrificial altar on which the victim priests and priestesses stand round, the temple sleep is induced and the sacrificial knife plunged in' (*British Homeopathic Journal* [1974], 63, 82).

But in searching for hidden meanings I would like to draw on psychoanalysis and anthropology in order to make a comparison between 'primitive' society and our own. In looking through the literature on the subject I am impressed by the relative lack of work on the interpretation of childbirth. It seems to me that the two studies of most interest are neither of recent origin: that of the anthropologist Van Gennep[3] and the psychoanalyst Reik.[4] In summarizing these studies I shall make use of an earlier paper.[5]

Van Gennep's Interpretation of Childbirth

Arnold Van Gennep published *Les rites de passage* in 1909. In this work he attempted to show that the ceremonies which attach to certain life-crises are similar in having the function of easing the transition from one state to the next and he used the term 'rite of passage' to describe the practices which occur when any barrier, physical, biological, or social, has to be crossed. He shows that, to a greater or lesser degree, such ceremonies can be divided into three stages: separation, transition, and incorporation. The ceremonies that are performed are done so with the purpose of separating the person from his previous state, nursing him through a transitional period, and finally incorporating him into the class of persons of which he is to become a member.
In his introduction to the 1960 (the first English) translation of Van Gennep's work, Kimball writes:

> Van Gennep, with others, accepted the dichotomy of the sacred and the profane; in fact, this is a central concept for understanding the transitional stage in which an individual or group finds itself from time to time. The sacred is not an absolute value but one relative to the situation. The person who enters a state at variance with the one previously held becomes 'sacred' to the others who remain in the profane stage. It is this new condition which calls for rights eventually incorporating the individual into the group and returning him to the customary routines of life. These changes may be dangerous, and, at the least, they are upsetting to the life of the group and the individual. The transitional period is met with rites of passage which cushion the disturbance. In one sense, all life is transition, with rhythmic periods of quiescence and heightened activity.

Certain features of Van Gennep's interpretation are immediately apparent:

1. Childbirth ritual has no distinctive characteristic over and above those to be observed in other rites of passage;

An Interpretation of Modern Obstetric Practice   195

2. The ritualistic feature that his theory is best suited to explain is the segregation of the parturient mother;
3. Ritual serves to ease change which is conceived as being extremely difficult for individual and society; it has a directly positive, beneficial function which, although of unspecified origin, is implicitly attributed to the society as a whole;
4. The actors are the individual and society and little mention is made of the needs and aims of the family.

Van Gennep's interpretation has relevance not only to the segregation of the mother but to the notions of purity and pollution which surround childbirth in so many societies, including our own. The explanations given by contemporary medicine for the control of contagion are simply inadequate. In a study of the use of masks and other protective clothing in a hospital for tuberculosis Roth[6] found that the occasions when staff and patients were required to wear masks had less to do with the actual risk of infection than with extraneous factors, including staff hierarchy. His report gives confirmation to the suggestion I make in chapter 14 that patients in hospital, whether sick or parturient, are subject to a taboo because they are in an uncertain and ambiguous state which cannot be readily accommodated by a highly ordered society. In that chapter I make the further suggestion (relevant to the discussion below) that illness engenders a painful inequality of power which may provoke exploitation either by patient or society, for which crisis taboo is a crude emergency method of control.

Reik's Interpretation of Childbirth

In contradistinction to Van Gennep—and following where Freud[7] had led—Theodore Reik is not content to regard rites of passage as practices organized by society for the benefit of the individual but view them primarily as manifestations of ambivalence to the initiate. In reference to couvade he writes:

> The prohibition of the realization of hostile wishes towards his wife, which the primitive man has imposed upon himself, exceeds the period of her confinement because his conconscious wishes continue to press towards active expression through the motor system. The temptation to realize these wishes is not overcome; it is merely displaced, and the protective measures against it have also to move with it. This keeping the man in bed has also the object of protecting his wife from his sexual and hostile wishes. Although up to now we have especially emphasised the pripondering share of aggressive tendencies in the building up of couvade, it must

not be forgotten that by means of them an inhibition of sexual wishes may arise .... His inhibited libido joins itself to those inborn sadistic instinctual components which the woman's condition brings to the fore and is turned into latent hate against her. Wicked desires now awaken towards the pregnant woman for whose body the man longs and which is forbidden to him.

Reik sees the protective magic which the husband undertakes on behalf of his wife—the warding-off of devils—as an act of reparation, an attempt to counteract his own projected hostility. Dietetic couvade is viewed—in an similar light—as a reaction-formation against the unconscious desire to devour the baby. What is the reason for this unconscious hostility towards the wife and baby? According to Reik it is primarily rooted in the Oedipus complex. The custom of the sacrifice of the firstborn male is, in Reik's view, a consequence of the same fantasy; the infant is sacrificed to the father (God) to assuage Oedipal guilt, a procedure which has the added advantage of eliminating the Oedipal rival of the next generation.

The Question of Envy

Although Reik is convincing in showing us the husband's repressed hostility and his manoeuvres to counteract it, the reasons for the hostility are not so clearly demonstrated. Is the Oedipus complex the only explanation, or even the most obvious one? If the father's fantasy is that 'it is not the mother who has given birth to the child but the father; to him therefore the child's love must go,' the simplest explanation for such a wish is that he wanted to create the child himself and to experience the child's love for him.

Crawley[8] has expressed the view that theories of marriage and birth customs 'show a sympathy with the father and with the child, but forget the mother, and are thus a modern document, illustrating the history of woman's treatment by man.' It would seem that Reik falls into the error which Crawley impugns to his predecessor. His theory is male-centred and this shows itself first in his failure to conceive that maternity could be an enviable state, and, secondly, that he leaves the woman's psychology out of the thesis.

The psychoanalyst Melanie Klein has stressed the envy which exists in relation to female creativity, and although her ideas about the origin and theoretical implications of envy are open to question, the clinical material that she has adduced is convincing. In chapter 10 I have brought evidence to suggest that a parturient mother does, in fact, expect to be envied, and that a dread of such envy may contribute to her mental breakdown. In his book *Symbolic Wounds: Puberty Rites and the Envious Male* Bettleheim[9] surveys the initiation ceremony of puberty and concludes that a neglected aspect of its meaning centres on male envy. He believes that there is a crucial difference between male and female circumcision: 'That women can bear children is taken for granted—it is demonstrable. Only men have to participate in ritual rebirth drama.' And the wounds inflicted at puberty spring from the wish to menstruate. By contrast there is a 'relative absence of ceremony accompanying female circumcision.' He suggests that female circumcision is imposed by men on girls in order 'to gain understanding of or power over the process of female genital bleeding' and 'as an expression of their anger at and envy of women's ability to bear children when men cannot.' In reference to couvade he writes: 'the man who is envious of the woman's ability to bear children has no "sympathy" for her. She is expected, if not compelled, to resume her work immediately, though she is exhausted from labour and the physiological readjustments. The husband and father, on the other hand, rests. His empathy with the mother is so great that he recreates in himself the need for special care that would be appropriate and that he denies to her.' Bettelheim thereby focuses on a central feature of childbirth ritual, and one that is mirrored in the way in which the ritual has been interpreted by our society; it is Hamlet without the Prince.*

Envy of maternity is now, however, confined to the male. Although the evil spirits which need to be propitiated by various actions performed as part of childbirth ritual are not, for the most part, specifically male; there exists a vast mythology surrounding female beings who do not take kindly to the event of childbirth; namely witches. Witches are said to cause sterility, abortion, and to steal, kill, or eat newborn babies; and, although they possess certain phallic features,

---

* In her paper 'Couvade and menstruation' Mary Douglas[10] criticises Bettelheim's thesis on the grounds that, improperly, he interprets public ritual in the light of his experiences with individual psychopathology, and she maintains that the explanation of the former must be in terms of the structure of the particular society in which it appears. This is a criticism with which psychoanalysts must now be familiar. But a way seems open for recognizing that the discrepancy is not so wide as it appears, for sexual envy and social imbalance (as Douglas, up to a point, suggests) may both occur in the same society and have a direct bearing on each other.

they are women, and themselves childless—they only have cats. Moreover they are old; perhaps what they envy most is youth (and what is younger than a newborn baby?). It would seem possible that the belief in witches arises first from the fact that such women—even if less exotic than those portrayed in myth—do exist in reality, and, secondly, from the projections of the parturient mother herself. Such projections in turn probably have a dual origin; the mother's hostile, envious, and condemning mother-image and her own unconscious hostility towards her baby (it is to be noted that the eating taboos of 'dietetic couvade' are not restricted to the male).

The Psychology of the Mother

It can be seen from the above description that childbirth customs in our society bear a definite similarity in certain respects to the ancient birth rituals, notably in the practice of segregating the mother and transferring the significance of the procedure away from her. In couvade the husband is significant; in our society one sometimes has the impression that it is the doctor; and the degree by which he takes control of her function—even the details of procedure such as ritual shaving and periotomy—put one in mind of female circumcision and Bettelheim's interpretation of this as an attempt on the part of the male to master his envy. And it would seem that, in general, the interpretations he makes about primitive society are equally applicable to our own; moreover, this similarity of pattern, despite the difference in social structure and rationale, adds weight to the interpretation.

I have mentioned that the interpretations of birth ritual so far made have excluded one notable item: the psychology of the mother. Although, as suggested above, this probably in some measure stems from a bias on the part of the interpreters it must be confessed that the reported facts left them little to go on. Because the mother plays an unspectacular part in the events she does not reveal her mind. In studying our own culture we are in a better position because we can ask her about it.

If it is true that the mother has been cast into a passive, even humiliating, role, it is one which she appears to accept readily. The labour and lying-in wards are not scenes of revolt, and the mother accepts the views, attitudes, and commands of her advisors with meekness. She does not violently claim her baby when he is taken from her

An Interpretation of Modern Obstetric Practice

and left to cry in another room. Many mothers, on the contrary, not only accept the regime but welcome it, preferring to be delivered under cover of anaesthesia, to leave the responsibility of nursing the baby to others and to substitute the bottle for breast. But we should not be persuaded by her submissiveness or even overt embracement of her situation into believing it is a genuine and natural wish. Not only is she confronted with the problem of opposing a powerful social force, but, if the argument put forward above has some validity, she will be subject to masochistic urges to propitiate.

A source of confusion over this question lies in the tendency to regard the cultural norms as the biologically necessary. In chapter 12 I have attempted to show that one characteristic of the mother in our society regarded by common consent and by psychoanalytical theory to be normal, yet in fact pathological and crippling both to herself and her child, is masochism. Psychotherapeutic investigation of mothers suffering from postpartum breakdown reveals the existence of such an urge, originating in guilt feelings and fear of envy is not necessarily a neurotic one—nor confined to mothers who break down—but one based on an unhappy reality which causes her to propitiate those around her by making costly sacrifices?

Summary

My aim in writing this chapter is to suggest some ways in which the rationale of current childbirth care is open to question. In the first place, we may be so under the influence of the overt organizational-technological viewpoint that we take a rather limited look at the over-all needs of mother, baby, and family. In the second place, there would appear to be hidden, underlying patterns in society which influence the way we handle childbirth. These two factors are not independent of each other. For instance, the drive to control childbirth by technical measures, a drive which seems to reach obsessive dimensions at times, may derive some of its force from unconscious feelings of antipathy towards the process of procreation.

A comparison with childbirth ritual in primitive society suggests that our own practice may contain elements, both positive and negative, the reasons for which we are largely unaware. We offer the mother a *rite de passage*, a period of respite from the demands of everyday life, during which she can effect the difficult transition of childbirth and nursing. But we do not allow her much time for this change and our means of helping her is to take her to a place where she is subjected to excessive control and where the spontaneous, loving relationship between mother and baby, so vital to the future development of both, is all too often made difficult or impossible. Indeed the degree of her subordination is so great that one wonders if the *rite de passage* serves to facilitate control in a way that is far less advantageous to the mother (at least in our own society) than the ideas of Van Gennep would suggest.

In searching for possible means for the existence of a concealed hostility to childbirth which limits our capacity to help the mother and child one could think in terms of the conflict between men and women, individual and state, or physical and spiritual. But the conflict which has, I believe, the deepest significance, is that between creativity and sterility.

Both society and the individual maintain their liveliness by a compromise between stasis and growth. It would appear that, in the forms in which we know them, growth presents them with a problem that is difficult and dangerous and from which they project themselves with a greater or lesser degree of rigidity. To the extent that this occurs, they fear growth and change. Certainly the conservative element in society is a very powerful one and it is no doubt this fact that has led to the 'functionalist' theory of social systems, of which that of Talcott Parsons is an influential descendant. The distrust and alarm with which manifestations of creativity in art, science, or religion is met is impressive, and adults do not take easily to the spontaneous creativity and innocent penetration of the child. Is it not then to be expected that the creative event of birth will be viewed with a similar degree of anxiety? A mother and baby are very appropriate symbols of growth, and for this reason a rigid and insecure society may see the necessity to control and restrict their spontaneous joy. Just as plants will manage to grow in the cracks between paving stones, so does joy emerge in our labour wards, but this fact should not diminish our efforts to seek out whatever stands in its way.

References

1. Illich, I. (1975), *Medical Nemesis*, Calder & Boyars, London.
2. Cohen, A. (1974), *Two-Dimensional Man*, Routledge & Kegan Paul, London.
3. Van Gennep, A. (1960), *The Rites of Passage*, Routledge & Kegan Paul, London.
4. Reik, T. [1914] 1962, 'Couvade and Fear of Retaliation,' in *Ritual: Four Psychoanalytic Studies*, Grove Press, New York.
5. Lomas, P. (1966), 'Ritualistic Elements in the Management of Childbirth,' *British J. of Med. Psychol.* 39, p. 207.
6. Roth, J. (1963), 'Ritual and Magic in the Control of Contagion,' *Amer. Sociol.* 22, p. 310.
7. Freud, S. (1913), 'Totem and Taboo,' in *The Complete Psychological Works of Sigmund Freud*, Hogarth, London.
8. Crawley, E. (1927), *The Mystic Rose*, 2d ed., Methuen, London.
9. Bettelheim, B. (1955), *Symbolic Wounds*, Thames & Hudson, London.
10. Douglas, M. (1968), 'Couvade and Menstruation,' in *Implicit Meanings*, edited by M. Douglas, Routledge & Kegan Paul, London.

14

Taboo and Illness

The purpose of this chapter is twofold: first, to make a reappraisal of the concept of taboo in the light of both psychoanalytic and anthropological writings on the subject; second, to consider the taboos surrounding illness in our society in the hope thereby of shedding some light both on the nature of taboo and the complexity of our response to illness.

There are several reasons why social anthropologists have been so unreceptive to Freud's work on taboo: (1) the section of *Totem and Taboo*[1] which has attracted the most attention from critics is that in which Freud imaginatively reconstructs an act of parricide committed by a primitive horde in the remote past—one of the least defensible of his ideas; (2) Freud was an armchair anthropologist; he did not obtain his material firsthand and failed to take into account the particular social structure of the societies he studied; and (3) in equating the behaviour of primitive society with that of children and neurotics Freud took up a position which would now be criticised on the grounds that, in the first place, society and individual are not comparable entities, and secondly, the evolutionary social theory of Frazer (which Freud adopted) underestimates the sophistication of the 'primitive' mind.

Despite these errors (which are, for the most part, those of his generation) did Freud manage to say something valid and important about the nature of taboo? The main presentation of his ideas on the subject appeared in 'Taboo and Emotional Ambivalence,' the second of the four essays which comprise the book *Totem and Taboo*. He asserted that taboo comes into being whenever there is a desire to transgress a prohibition. 'The dangerous attribute of taboo,' he wrote, 'is the quality of exciting men's ambivalence and *tempting* them to transgress the prohibition.' The transgressor himself becomes infected by the taboo since 'he possesses the dangerous quality of tempting other to follow his example: why *should* he be allowed to do what is forbidden to others? *But,*

> a person who has not violated any taboo may yet be permanently or temporarily tabooed because he is in a state which possesses the quality of arousing forbidden desires in others and of awakening a conflict of ambivalence in them. The majority of exceptional states and exceptional positions are of this kind and possess this dangerous power. The king or chief arouses envy on account of his privileges: everyone, perhaps, would like to be a king. Dead men, newborn babies, and women menstruating or in labour stimulate desire by their special helplessness. . . .

Without effective taboos of this kind there would be a 'dissolution of the community.'

Some of Freud's examples may not be entirely correct—for instance, he was not able to conceive that childbirth could be an enviable state and thus attract taboo—but his account of the categories would seem to be valid. It perhaps needs to be noted that the helpless person is liable to be in a state of envy and thus may be considered revengeful and inherently dangerous—as Freud himself notes in his observations on the taboo of the dead—and therefore potential disrupters of the peace.

Freud's theory of taboo implies the view that whenever inequality of sufficient degree to arouse serious envy exists within a community, taboo helps to ensure against violent attempts to dissolve the inequality. To the extent that inequality is inherent in social systems—insofar as society is hierarchical—taboo is designed to maintain the social order: it is conservative in nature. Thus the persons selected for taboo are those of superior status (who may thereby provoke attack), those of inferior status (who may either provoke, by their helplessness, further humiliation and therefore inequality, or may launch a revengeful assault on their superiors), and those who, in breaking the taboo, have made a move in the direction of the feared disruption.

Freud believed that the effectiveness of taboo depends on the fact that it places vulnerable people out of harm's way: the enviable mighty and the weak. It would seem, however, that a slightly different explanation would account for the facts more adequately: that taboo works by accentuating the difference in status between the two classes in such a way that challenge is inconceivable. In this view taboo is a form of unconscious propaganda, a method of influencing belief rather than directly ensuring physical protection. The message it conveys is not 'This or that class of persons is sacred (or unclean),' but 'This class of person is sacred, whereas that class is unclean.' The confusion between sacred and unclean noted by Freud perhaps arises, first, because both the sacred and the unclean classes are tabooed by the same stroke (since the function of the taboo is to make a contrast it cannot evaluate one without the other), and secondly, on account of a counteracting tendency (presumably emanating from the weak) to reverse the judgement. That the aim of taboo in regard to the weak is not so altruistic as Freud believed is suggested by the fact that if the 'weak' class of persons tabooed is taken, as would be logical, to consist not only the helpless who might be exploited but all those outsiders—witches, strangers, tramps, criminals, and so forth—who might well be considered, owing to their dissatisfaction, immorality or novelty of ideas, a potential menace to the established order. Freud's suggestion—that one reason for the taboo on the dead was the fear that, being envious of the living, they are liable to come back to haunt the latter—is in keeping with this view.

It may be thought that incest taboos, being concerned with the restriction of sexual impulses, cannot be explained in this kind of way. However, whether the taboo is considered to derive from the set-up of the individual family or from inherited guilt over a social event in the distant past, it is clear that a question of status is involved: who is to be the head of the family or clan (as symbolised, among other things, by sexual domination)? The incest taboo is upon the generations: it reinforces and exaggerates the differences between them.

In his interpretation of phenomena, whether dreams, symptoms, myths, or works of art, Freud relies mainly on his conception of the unconscious, and his understanding of taboo is no exception. He draws attention to the fact that the origin of the taboo is unknown, and suggests that the reason for this is that some part of the emotion aroused by the tabooed person is too painful to be admitted to consciousness. The suggestion that taboo may also be a form of propaganda gives another reason for its meaning remaining unknown—the need for those who set themselves up as sacred to conceal both their human frailty and the fact that they are aiming at power. It does not follow that they themselves remain unaware of the true situation, but perhaps, in order to enhance their sense of importance and relieve the guilt which might result from cynical indulgence in brainwashing techniques, they usually achieve a high degree of self-deception.

However, as Jones[2] showed, an idea may remain unconscious not only because it is objectionable but because there is no other way in which it can (yet) be formulated. It is by a similar formula that Langer bases her study of myth, ritual and art. She writes:

> The origin of myth is dynamic, but its purpose is philosophical. It is the primitive phase of metaphysical thought, the first embodiment of *general ideas*. It can do no more than initiate and present them; for it is a non-discursive symbolism, it does not lend itself to analytic and genuinely abstractive techniques.[3]

Insofar as this line of thought is applicable to taboo, it would seem that the latter is the best formula that society can find, in some circumstances, to provide an understanding and maintenance of the structure of society; it is a crude homeostatic principle, concerned with the balance of power.

Van Gennep's Interpretation

Although taboo in primitive society has been extensively documented in the literature of social anthropology only a few attempts have been made to understand the meaning of the concept. The two most useful formulations that I can find are by Van Gennep[4] and Douglas.[5]

Van Gennep believed that the taboo which is imposed upon the person in a state of transition has the function of easing his passage; it separates him from his previous state, protects him during the transitional period and introduces him into his newly acquired social position. For this reason taboo is prominent in the major changes of the life-cycle: birth, puberty, marriage, parenthood, and death. It can be seen that taboo, according to Van Gennep, has the function of preserving the social hierarchy, but, unlike the interpretation which I have derived from Freud, it does so not by maintaining the rigid separation of people into their respective social categories but by enabling them to make a transition from one category to another with the least possible disturbance to themselves and society. Van Gennep's formulation deals with the person who is in a rather similar situation to the one who transgresses a taboo, but who, unlike the latter, is permitted to do so—and this would seem to be the point. Insofar as the transition is socially acceptable, taboo facilitates it, if it is regarded as an illegitimate transgression, taboo reinforces the prohibition. However, the manner in which initiation ceremonies are conducted in primitive societies—and, as suggested in the previous chapter, the way in which childbirth is managed in our own society—suggests that, although there is an element of helpfulness towards the initiate, the latter is subjected to unnecessary control and humiliation, a phenomenon which betrays the reluctance with which those in authority permit the inevitable entrance of a newcomer to their midst. Thus, despite the fact that Van Gennep's view introduces the interesting idea that taboo may be concerned not only with the rigid maintenance of social structure but with change and progression, its function is perhaps more akin to that of a subtle but reactionary administrator, who aims to limit change to the minimum possible without provoking a revolution.

Douglas's Interpretation

Unlike most social anthropologists, Douglas records the fact that her own personal reflections on the subject (particularly in relation to dirt) have played a part in the formulation of her theory. This is significant in that one of the differences between the approach of the psychoanalyst and that of the anthropologist is that the former starts from observations of individuals and draws conclusions about social forms, while the latter analyses the structure of society with little reference to the motives of the individual of which it consists—each worker risking a one-sided view. In the main, however, Douglas relies on the analysis of social structure; in doing so she possesses a knowledge of data, obtained from the field studies of recent years, of a more reliable kind than that available to Freud or Van Gennep.

Douglas concludes that taboo reinforces social conformity:

> Political power is usually held precariously and primitive rulers are no exception. So we find their legitimate pretensions backed by beliefs in extraordinary powers emanating from their persons—from the insignia of their office or from words they can utter. Similarly the ideal order of society is guarded by dangers which threaten

transgressors. These danger-beliefs are as much threats which one man uses to coerce another as dangers which he himself fears to incur by his own lapses from righteousness.

Thus Douglas conceives that an important function of taboo is the maintenance of social (and particularly hierarchical) order. She notes that taboo arises at points of uncertainty, that

> people really do think of their own environment as consisting of other people joined or separated by lines which must be respected . . . ; [and that] wherever the lines are precarious we find that pollution ideas come into their own.

Although she arrives, by a much more straightforward route than that outlined above, at the notion that taboo is, or at least can be, a form of propaganda, and she illuminates many details of the symbolic transformations of taboo, Douglas does not, to my mind, satisfactorily explain the reason why taboo has to operate in such devious ways; and this is because she completely ignores unconscious factors. One wonders, for instance, *why* certain lines of communication are precarious? Is it because it would be too painful or dangerous to bring the truth clearly into the open?

> Dirt [maintains Douglas] was created by the differentiating activity of mind; it was a by-product of the creation of order. So it started from a state of non-differentiation; all through the process of differentiating its role was to threaten the distinctions made; finally it returns to its true indiscriminable character . . . In its last phase then, dirt shows itself as an apt symbol of creative formlessness. But it is from its first phase that it derives its force. The danger which is risked by boundary transgression is power. Those vulnerable margins and those attacking forces which threaten to destroy good order represent the powers inherent in the cosmos.

It is a convincing idea that taboo, although concerned with power and social order, is so often expressed in terms of the avoidance of pollution because dirt is an apt symbol of threatening 'creative formlessness' and finds a link with the psychoanalytic observation of the relation between anal fantasy and artistic creativity. Moreover, it is precisely the unstructured which is ambiguous—it may be a waste-product or a precious source of material, the thought of an imbecile or a genius—and which cannot be dealt with by logical means: taboo is itself an ambiguous reaction to it, making it possible to take some kind of illogical action or even (if one can make a generalisation from Van Gennep's theory) a means of holding the structure intact until the new entity can be absorbed safely.

Taboo in Our Society

Modern Western society has developed different methods of achieving the results for which taboo is used in primitive society: taboo has, as it were, become secularised. It appears to us to be of only marginal importance in holding society together now that we have a well-developed legal system and that the breaking of a taboo does not incur such dire penalties. But perhaps taboo is more of a force in the community than we realise. There are still examples of taboo—such as apartheid—which can have as far-reaching effects as those of primitive cultures. What is perhaps significant about our society in this respect is that we organise our rationalisations of taboo to a greater extent than primitive society and, because they are our own rationalisations, we are more readily convinced by them. One particularly effective rationalisation which we possess—and which I have not heard of in the literature on primitive society—is denial of the existence of the taboo in question. We are inclined to say, for instance, that nowadays there is no taboo on death, that death can be spoken about openly. But the taboo remains a full appreciation and expression of emotion about death. As an example of the way in which taboo works in our society, I shall consider the handling of illness.

The Taboo on Illness

In our society the sick are segregated. I do not only mean by this that they are put into a special place (a hospital) but that in the process of transportation a threshold is crossed of greater significance than the hospital door and that they enter a different class of persons. The patient loses status and autonomy, and contact with previous social attachments is discouraged. They become subject to the authority of a person (the doctor) with very high prestige, before whom they are obliged to humble themselves. The force behind this pattern is a very strong one and it has taken, and continues to take, remarkable tenacity on the part of those reformers aware of the psychological disadvantages to the patient of this tradition in order to make changes. (I think, for instance, of the drive to allow mothers to visit and look after their children in hospital). What is the origin of this system of behaviour?
To some extent segregation and control of the patient are natural and reasonable. He can be observed and medically treated more effec-

tively, protected from the possible harmful activity of himself or others, and prevented from passing on his illness to others (in the case of infection) or being too great a burden and anxiety to them. But these measures have been carried out, at least until recently, with much greater rigidity and force than is warranted or reasonable: the paraphernalia which surrounded the consultant's ward round, the treatment of the patient as someone of low intelligence and sensitivity (not a full human being), and the jargon and secrecy of medical notes. Moreover, the degree to which the patient was segregated and dehumanised varies according to the severity of the illness in a way that cannot be explained simply as measures of necessary medical treatment. The more disabling, disfiguring, chronic, inexplicable, uncontrollable the illness the greater the person is held in horror and the greater the distance placed between himself and others. Those diseases associated with hereditary taint are particularly liable to arouse this kind of attitude, a fact which, at present, influences social approaches to the radiation victims of Hiroshima. But perhaps the attitude reaches it height in the case of mental illness, as is made vividly clear by Goffman's[7] account of life in a mental hospital from the patient's viewpoint. What are the forces which bring about this pattern?

A likely explanation is that a taboo is in operation which segregates the healthy from the sick. The patient is first separated from the community, then a further separation is made between him and his caretaker (the doctor), who, however, being attributed with semi-magical powers—being himself taboo—can deal with this dangerous person. Why is the sick man dangerous? The answer would seem to be that he is dangerous because he is in a weak position: his illness has engendered a painful inequality which may arouse passions and provoke exploitation by either patient or society. Those around him may wish to crush him as a nuisance in practice, a reminder of mortality, a demand on love and tolerance which perhaps they do not possess, and a disgrace to the family (especially in the case of a disease considered to be hereditary); he in turn may feel hate and envy of the healthy, and may attempt to use his weakness, judo style, in order to gain dominance. A hierarchy has developed between him and those around him, between the weak and the strong. Taboo is an attempt on the part of the community to confront this predicament with the minimum of disruption. It is a crude method for dealing with an emergency, a method which has worked in a fashion at enormous cost.

Illness, however, is a complex state and not simply a condition of disability. It may, in certain circumstances, be entered into during a period of change or growth as one possible means of negotiating the transition, a fact which is most clearly evident in the case of psychological illness. It was the discovery of Freud that the symptom has meaning, and the positive, creative aspects of mental disorder have been explored by several psychoanalysts, notably Erikson[8] and Winnicott.[9] That physical illness may sometimes similarly be an atypical manifestation of growth—not only in children—is perhaps an observation more easily available to the general practitioner than the psychiatrist. I suspect that many cases of 'post-infective' depression or debility arise from a person's need to become ill or to use an accidental illness for the purpose of making a necessary psychological (and possibly physical) change. In practice, such attempts risk failure because their true meaning is unrecognized by the doctor.

The function of the taboo on illness in such a case is to allow the patient to separate himself from the demands of the community to conform; it allows him to wrench himself away from an identity which has come to be expected of him and in which he has become cramped; it holds together the relationship between patient and society until he can be assimilated again in his changed state. In this aspect of its function the taboo on illness is similar to that imposed upon pubescence and parturition.

Illness, therefore, is an ambiguous state, as are all states subject to taboo, and society, with its dual loyalty to the group and the individual, to change and conservation, to creativity and conformity, is inevitably ambivalent towards the sick person. This ambivalence is a feature of a contemporary debate which arouses some heat in the psychiatric world: that of the existence and nature of mental illness. On the one hand, there is the traditional psychiatric view of the patient as a person who is simply disabled, who has something wrong with him which needs to be rectified in order that he may match up to the rest of the population. On the other hand is the more recent assertion, put forward by writers arguing from entirely different standpoints, such as Szasz[10] and Laing,[11] that mental illness does not exist. Whereas Szasz regards it as a myth propagated by the patient for his own benefit, Laing views it as a myth propagated by society for its own sake. One feels that the contemporary (anti-psychiatric) view has arisen out of need to show that mental illness is not a fixed unambiguous state of disability, as has been previously thought, but a state embraced by a person, whether for constructive or destructive purposes, in order to oppose the values and forces around him. The proponents of this conception tend to defend the point of view either of the patient or society, but this preoccupation obscures their assertion that acute mental illness constitutes an attempt at change. It would seem to be a distortion of language to say that mental illness does not exist—the person is disabled in the sort of way that we commonly mean when we say that someone is ill—but the fact of disability is not necessarily the most important part of his state; his illness may incorporate important aims to which disability is a necessary, if painful, dangerous and disruptive, side effect. The crude, makeshift approach of taboo may allow the person in such a predicament some leeway, may give sufficient temporary breathing space, for him to make the necessary change, but, while the nature of illness remains obscure and an ambivalence flourishes undetected in our methods of dealing with the sick, it can only give very inadequate provision for him.

Conclusion

In comparing the taboos of primitive society with those he observed in the behaviour of his obsessional patients Freud concluded that both were a consequence of an infantile level of development—and in this he was mistaken. But with the intuitive genius that so often enabled him to get at the core of the matter, even when his data and his reasoning were at fault, his comparison was a valid one. Taboo is a nondiscursive means of avoiding confusion—intrapsychic, interpersonal, and societal. It is a method of keeping apart incompatible elements when the reason for doing so eludes conscious thought.

The importance of taboo is not confined to primitive society but exists in several areas of our own society—of which illness is one—being masked by rationalizations. Illness is an ambiguous state partly because the degree to which it is motivated or enforced is usually uncertain and partly because it involves a change of status provoking emotions of shame, hate, pity, envy, and despair which must remain unconscious. There is no well-organised system—such as the legal system envisaged by Samuel Butler in *Erewhon*—for separating incompatibles (the sick and the well), so taboo has to fill the gap.

Although taboo exists for the benefit of both the individual and society, it is open to abuse by both. In the field of illness—particularly mental illness—it may be used by the healthy to maintain a position of power and by both the healthy and the sick to avoid responsibility.

References

1. Freud, S. (1913), 'Totem and Taboo,' in *The Complete Psychological Works of Sigmund Freud*, Hogarth, London.
2. Jones, E. (1913), 'The Theory of Symbolisms,' in *Papers on Psychoanalysis*, Wood, New York.
3. Langer, S. (1960), *Philosophy in a New Key*, Harvard University Press, Cambridge, MA.
4. Van Gennep, A. (1960), *Les rites de passage*, Routledge & Kegan Paul, London.
5. Douglas, M. (1966), *Purity and Danger*, Routledge & Kegan Paul, London.
6. Lifton, R.J. (1964), 'On Death and Death Symbolism: The Hiroshima Disaster,' *Psychiatry* 27, pp. 181–210.
7. Goffman, E. (1961), *Asylums*, Doubleday, New York.
8. Erikson, E. (1959), *Identity and the Life Cycle*, International Universities Press, New York.
9. Winnincott, D.W. (1958), *Collected Papers*, Tavistock, London.
10. Szasz, T. (1961), *The Myth of Mental Illness*, Hoeber-Harper, New York.
11. Laing, R.D. (1960), *The Divided Self*, Tavistock, London.

15

Psychoanalysis—Freudian or Existential

I do not commonly like to regard myself as a Freudian because it implies certain things—that I am an atheist, a pessimist, that I insist that my patients lie on the couch, that I think in terms of id, ego, superego, and so forth—which, to my mind, are not essential to the practice of psychoanalysis. My only claim to the title is that I have received a training at a psychoanalytical institute, that I practice a method of therapy which bears a distinct resemblance to that advocated by Freud, and that I have not discovered any other label to stick on myself except the generic term 'psychotherapist.' And I hope to imply throughout this essay a condemnation of the type of thinking that freezes people into Freudian, Existential, or any other blocks of ice.

Freud grew up intellectually in the philosophical tradition of late nineteenth-century scientific materialism. It is often forgotten that his first contribution was to neurology—that is to say, it was in the field of physical medicine. When he turned his attention to psychology, he couched his earliest formulations—in his unpublished 'Project' discussed by Ernest Jones[1]—in neurological terminology, and when, later, in The Interpretation of Dreams,[2] he proposed the psychological theory that has formed the basis of psychoanalytical thinking, he uses a conceptual framework which markedly resembles the earlier one even though the references to physical structure are no longer there. Freud's

---

Published in *Psychoanalysis Observed,* editor, Rycroft, L., Constable, London, 1966.

failure to emancipate himself from the physical frame of thought has put psychoanalysis into a dilemma of which some practitioners are now becoming aware.

In 1964 Home read a paper to the British Psychoanalytical Society[3] which began with the passage:

> Psychoanalysis began as a study of neurosis and as an hypothesis explaining its origin and development. As an hypothesis about neurosis it might have made little enough stir, in spite of its delineation of an aetiology linking neurosis with sexual frustration, had Freud not invoked a totally new principle of explanation. This principle of explanation, which ran counter to the tenor of thought prevalent in medicine at the time, and which eventually led him on to formulate his revolutionary ideas about the unconscious mind, was that the symptom could have meaning.
> That the symptom has meaning, if it is neurotic, is Freud's basic discovery, the basic insight which opened up the way to an understanding of functional illness and the principles of psychoanalytic treatment. It is not surprising that, in the excitement of so great a discovery and one that opened up such vast new territories, Freud should have overlooked the logical implications for theory of the step he had taken. Those implications are, however, very great, for in the mechanistic medicine of Freud's time, as in all organic medicine of our own day, the symptom is logically regarded as a fact and a fact is regarded as the product of causes. In this, medicine simply follows the practice of chemico-physical science and the canons of thought which are exemplified with special clarity in physics. In discovering that the symptom had meaning and basing his treatment on this hypothesis, Freud took the psychoanalytic study of neurosis out of the world of science into the world of the humanities, because a meaning is not the product of causes but the creation of a subject. This is a major difference; for the logic and method of the humanities is radically different from that of science, though no less respectable and rational and of course much longer established.

The event described by Home has had ironic consequences. The man who, more than any other, has enabled us to see the mentally sick patient as more of a person and less of a thing than had hitherto been possible is now often discredited, especially by existentialists, as a reductionist and dehumaniser. That this has happened is largely due to the failure, outside the psychoanalytic movement, to recognize that Freud's findings transcend his language, and, by psychoanalysts themselves, to reformulate his findings in more worthy terms. Home is, alas, the exception and not the rule, and most psychoanalysts do not even recognize the pressing need for such a radical reformulation.

Currently, the psychoanalytic theory which holds the field goes by the name of 'ego psychology' and its leading exponent is Heinz Hartmann.[4] Freud's theory of instinctual drive and his structural model of id, ego, and superego is retained, but a much greater importance is attached to the ego than before. Psychoanalysts have become concerned with questions about the nature of 'self' and 'identity' and some valuable work has been done, notably by Erik Erikson[5] in this area of study, but the problem has arisen as to how to bridge the theoretical gap between these new interests and 'ego psychology.' The 'ego' is not the 'self'; it is a construct not an experience, it is mechanistic not personal, and it is alienated from its source of power, the 'id.' Attempts at reconciliation have produced the most ungainly and confused formulations.

What is psychoanalysis to do about this impasse? It is (in America, at least) a social force, it has a well-tried technique (psychoanalysts may adhere to a mechanistic theory, but fortunately they do not practise what they preach, as a perusal of their case-histories will show), and they have a vast clinical literature. Moreover, even confined by a theory that is basically askew, they have produced formulations about mental disharmony which no psychotherapist could ignore without the utmost peril. What must be retained and what should be scrapped? And—relevant to our theme—where does existentialism come in?

Existential analysis, jointly inspired by the work of Freud and the writings of the existentialist philosophers (notably Kierkegaard and Heidegger), had its main authorship in Ludwig Binswanger, a contemporary of Freud's. Much of the writing—and perhaps of the thinking—has not travelled well into Anglo-Saxon countries, although in America Rollo May et al. translated key works and elucidated the concepts concerned in the influential book Existence in 1958.[6] And the work of Buber and Tillich has made its mark on American psychiatry.

Common to all these thinkers is the basic existential tenet, similar to that expressed by Home in the passage quoted above: the person is more than a thing and cannot be adequately formulated in the terminology of natural science.

Existential analysis, therefore, starts without the encumbrance of a system of psychology based on the physical sciences and views the person as a whole being, the agent of his actions. This does not mean that it has solved the ancient philosophical problem of free will versus determinism—or, one of its modern derivatives, the validity of the concept of unconscious thought—but it is a theory which has the pragmatic advantage of being more in accord with our day to day experience of living. The critique which follows has, I hope, some application to the movement as a whole, but I shall confine myself mainly to existentialism in England with which I am most familiar and in sympathy.

The Divided Self

In The Divided Self[7] Laing—who, although a trained psychoanalyst acknowledges his 'main intellectual indebtedness to the existential tradition'—uses this approach to criticize conventional psychiatric thinking with the conviction and lucidity unavailable to someone using the theoretical framework of orthodox psychoanalysis (an approach which enables him to make a similar criticism of behaviour therapy).

In a cogent analysis of an interview with a patient described by Kraepelin (who was primarily responsible for our present classification of mental disorder and who is sometimes referred to as the 'father of modern psychiatry') Laing shows that the psychiatrist is too preoccupied with categorizing the behaviour of the patient to notice that the 'psychotic' utterances of the latter are reasonable, if disguised, objections to being merely classified and not treated as a person. It is with the dilemma which confronts those who are treated—not only by psychiatrists, but by parents and others—as a thing rather than a person, and with the schizoid, alienated states which result from such treatment, that Laing is concerned, and, using the existential frame of reference, he is able to present a description of such states more readily comprehensible by, and enriching to, those patients who suffer this particular kind of existence than one given in psychoanalytic terminology.

He writes: 'A man may have a sense of his presence in the world as a real, alive, whole, and, in a temporal sense, continuous person . . . Such a basically ontologically secure person will encounter all the hazards of life, social, ethical, spiritual, biological, from a centrally firm sense of his own and other people's reality and identity.'

If life-experience has not been such as to enable the person to acquire this 'primary ontological security,' he is forced into a continuous struggle to maintain a sense of his own being; in this weak position he fears 'engulfment' by others, the 'implosion' of external reality, the 'petrification' of 'becoming no more than a thing in the world of the other.'

The total self, the 'embodied self,' faced with disadvantageous conditions, may split into two parts, a disembodied 'inner self,' felt by the person to be the real part of himself, and a 'false self,' embodied but dead and futile, which puts up a front of conformity to the world. Is Laing merely using a more vivid language than that of traditional psychiatry and psychoanalysis or is he producing a more accurate theory of schizoid states? How far has he departed from Freud? What relationship do his ideas have to those of Melanie Klein or Winnicott, two influential British psychoanalysts with whom he has sometimes been compared? An actual problem, interpreted in a Freudian and an existential way, may serve as an introduction to a discussion of the contrasting positions.

In his autobiography The House of Elrig[8] Gavin Maxwell describes two recurrent childhood nightmares 'of such dreadful intensity that each was like a death in itself.'

In the first dream, 'I was playing on the lawn at Tynewood with my sister, the house was behind me, and beyond the lawn was woodland, fringed with rhododendrons. It was a strange half-light, the kind of darkness at noon that may come with a freak thunderstorm or an eclipse of the sun. There were many daisies on the lawn, and I was holding one in my hand when something like the mouth of a gigantic cannon, a vast gaping circle of darkness, ringed with dull metal, loomed out of the trees and grew until there was room for nothing else but it. There was no action, no attempt on my part to escape, only the object itself and the ultimate extreme of fear.'

In the second dream, 'the whole of my vision was filled by a ceiling, an ordinary undecorated ceiling of a pale grey colour. On the surface of this, at the far left and close to the corner, was an object that never came into absolute focus; it appeared to be a short, dark leather strap like a dog collar. Nothing moved; as in the other dream, terror was in the object itself.'

Dreams are difficult enough to understand, even when the dreamer is present and can tell us his associations, and I do not propose to attempt a detailed exposition. A Freudian (or Kleinian) interpretation would focus on anxiety aroused by the instinctual urges, symbolized by items in the dreams, which are of such intensity as to threaten the ego of the child: the thunderstorm may be thought to refer to rage, the gigantic cannon to aggressive—phallic or infantile—'oral' urges. There is certainly, in the first dream, an impressive contrast between the gentle little boy, playing happily with his sister on the lawn, holding a daisy, and the crushing destructiveness of the cannon. Such contrasts are typical of the conflict between aggressive impulse and the 'reaction formation' against it.

But what of the circumstances of the dreams? Maxwell tells us that they reached their climax during his internment in a preparatory boarding school, a school passionately dedicated to the suppression of individuality in its pupils, the emotional atmosphere of which was even more chilling than the early morning cold showers which were a routine feature of the curriculum.

Shortly before this climax was reached Maxwell was admonished for using his own portable inkwell by a senior boy: 'You've got to learn to be like other people.' His subsequent attempt to assert his individuality in this matter failed ignominiously.

If one turns again to the dreams one can see that they both depict a situation of paralysis in the face of a crushing environment; the images—an 'eclipse of the sun,' a 'vast gaping darkness, ringed with dull metal . . . grew until there was room for nothing else but it,' a grey ceiling, a dog collar—these are images of constriction and oppression. The dreams depict, in fact, the actual situation of the boy, and it is upon this aspect that an existential approach would focus: the present predicament of the person (as a whole) in his immediate interpersonal relationships in the school—and also with his family who were responsible for sending him to the school.

These dreams were not analyzed, the services of no therapist were called upon, but the boy was cured—or rather, cured himself. Presumably because he retained sufficient belief in himself, in life, or in his mother's capacity to respond to an extreme appeal, he took desperate action which resulted in his removal from the school. Once removed, his peace of mind was restored and he prospered.

It would appear, therefore, that the second existential kind of interpretation of the dream is the more meaningful. It does not follow, however, that the first view is incorrect, or the second comprehensive. As Freud has shown, dreams are massively condensed structures. There is plenty of biographical evidence in Maxwell's book to suggest the existence of serious sexual and aggressive repression at the time of the dreams.

Melanie Klein

Melanie Klein[9] has made an enormous impression on the theory and practice of psychoanalysis in this country. Basing her ideas on child analysis—of which she was a pioneer—she held that the crucial period of life was infancy and that the innate aggressive tendencies of the baby led him early into intolerable conflict over love and hate from which he tried to escape by projecting the aggressive part of himself on the outer world.

Like Freud, she emphasized the disrupting effect of powerful instinctual drive, but she focused on the aggressive rather than the sexual drive and believed that the major conflict occurred at an even earlier age than did he. Although all of us, she held, carry the scars of this struggle, those destined to become 'schizoid' have been crippled by it.

The anxieties characteristic of the schizoid person, described by Laing as 'ontological insecurity,' 'a fear of engulfment,' etc., are discussed by Melanie Klein in terms of 'persecutory anxiety,' 'projective and introjective identification,' but the similarity of descriptive clinical detail is apparent. Both writers are impressed by the splitting mechanisms which occur, on feelings of inner deadness and impoverishment, on terror of an invasion into the very core of the self. But the agreement ends here. Laing believes that such a person is struggling to maintain his sense of identity in the face of a total life-experience designed to destroy it. Melanie Klein held the view that such insecurity arises from unrealistic fantasies of attack which in turn have their source in the person's projection of his aggression; this projection takes place in infancy in cases where there is an excess of aggression either innately determined or engendered by physical frustration, and is therefore experienced in terms of bodily fantasy, the mouth and breast having special significance.

Having myself come to view the nature of fears of 'engulfment' in a way rather similar to that of Laing, I must confess to a leaning towards his explanation and language. Melanie Klein, in fact, is no existentialist, but a true Freudian, deeply committed to instinct theory, almost blind to the life circumstances of the patient. Although she tried to develop a theory of interpersonal relationships (which, in psychoanalytical theory goes by the unfortunate term 'object relationships') she did not achieve the success of Fairbairn in this venture. Persons do not, in her thinking, ever really emerge from their internal fantasy world; love is not a spontaneous emotion but is based on a need to make reparation for aggressive wishes and fantasies. Her contribution lies not in basic theory but in her description of certain defence mechanisms. She has, for instance, extended our awareness of projection, revealing that not only aggression is projected but also other undesirable states of mind such as anxiety, guilt and depression, and that such projection is often accompanied by a massive identification, depleting to the self. That her work provoked such a furor within the psychoanalytic movement is surprising in view of its intrinsic significance, and is to be attributed to a combination of group intolerance and her own tendency to write somewhat dogmatically.

The difference between the Freudian and the existential viewpoint is therefore not bridged in any way by the work of Melanie Klein, for her position is essentially that of Freud. But this difference is not one of total incompatibility; there is no reason why both the intrusion of the environment and the projection of undesired emotional states should not combine in the production of symptoms. About the language used to describe the experiences of engulfment, etc., a further point needs to be added. If the schizoid person is encouraged—as he is by Laing—to formulate his anxieties in non-bodily, non-infantile language, may this not facilitate the idealization of conceptual thinking at the expense of bodily experience to which the schizoid person is rather prone?? Is there not a danger of forgetting that the original deprivations, even if best formulated in terms of 'self,' 'identity,' and so on, were to a large extent physical? However misguided was Freud's biological theory of human development it enabled him to remain aware at all times that we have bodies.

Winnicott

Like Melanie Klein, Winnicott derived many of his ideas from the psychoanalysis of children, but is more concerned than she with the actuality of the mother-baby relationship. He believes that it is a failure on the part of the mother to make meaningful contact with her baby that prevents him from revealing his 'true self' to her and forces him into a schizoid mould in which a 'false self' is presented to the world, leaving the 'true self' buried and unmanifest. The similarity of language to that of Laing in describing this alienated condition is clear, yet Winnicott does not appear to claim any kinship with the existential tradition.

Although much of Winnicott's thought stems from his work with mothers and babies, the paper in which he describes his theory of schizoid states is based on his observation of adult patients in the psychoanalytic setting.[10] His experience led him to believe that for certain patients it is necessary, at some point in the analysis, to give up a 'false' independence and regress to a state of 'real' dependence on the analyst, who may, at this stage, be called upon to 'hold' the patient in addition to performing his customary function of interpretation. If the outcome of this crisis is satisfactory the patient begins to trust the outer world; his 'true self' may then emerge, and grow.

In this conception the inner self is not only felt as more real by the patient but contains the germ of the 'true self,' 'frozen' at the time of the environmental failure, waiting to be awakened by a kinder world. The 'false self' not only conforms, in the meaningless way described by Laing, to the demands of the outer world, but acts as a 'caretaker' to the 'true self.' Apart from the fact that Winnicott is concerned with a therapeutic technique rather than a clinical or theoretical description of schizoid states, the main difference in his approach is his belief in the existence of a pre-split 'real' self to which one has to return. Like Laing, Winnicott focuses on the 'impingement' of a disruptive environment on a vulnerable self, but he places the critical time for this occurrence in infancy. He believes, as did Freud, that it is necessary in therapy to revive an early infantile memory. This does not mean that particular well-defined incidents need emerge from repression, but that there must be a return to the infantile experience of simple, passionate openness preceding the disappointment that led to withdrawal and splitting. Certain elements in Winnicott's terminology remain unsatisfactory, for he has tried to retain Freudian 'metapsychology' in parts of his description, and a clear distinction between the pre-split self, the 'false self,' and the distorted fantasy-system of the 'inner self' is lacking, but he conveys, even more vividly than Laing, the picture of a self that remains its own agent in any eventuality and however disguised, and he retains the conception—vital to psychoanalytic thought—of a return to the past. This last factor is of crucial importance in any discussion of the different viewpoints of Freudian and existential analysis.

The 'Unconscious'

One of the cornerstones of Freud's theory is 'unconsciousness,' a concept closely linked to 'repression' (of thoughts and feelings into the unconscious), to the 'transference' (of unconscious—particularly infantile—yearnings on to the analyst) and'resistance' (to acceptance of the emergent wishes and fears).

Existentialists are keenly critical about this concept. Sartre, in Being and Nothingness[11] demonstrates that the notion of 'unconsciousness' is in fact a contradiction in terms. A distinction must be made here between disagreements about the concept of 'the unconscious' and about the nature of that which the term denotes. As regards the former, one may accept that Freud's formulation of 'the unconscious' is unsatisfactory inasmuch as it gives the impression of an actual place in the mind into which things could be put. But there is no objection, except perhaps a semantic one, to his use of the term when describing certain experiences in psychoanalytic treatment (a fact which some existentialists, including Laing, accept). The illumination that occurs when a potential perception is made actual is an experience of everyday life carrying conviction, although seldom felt with the intensity with which it occurs in a psychotherapeutic setting. It would seem likely that an explanation of what makes it impossible to actualize a potential experience awaits resolution of the question as to what makes it possible. In the meantime we need the term (or some equivalent) just as we need the term 'free will' (or 'agency'), for which also there is no adequate conception.

Given this amount of agreement, there would appear to be no reason why existentialists should object to the concept of 'transference' of unconscious material onto the analyst, yet this concept is little mentioned in existential writings. The reason for this, I suspect, is partly a disagreement with Freud as to what is transferred, and partly the fear of an unhealthy preoccupation with the past. In psychoanalytical theory, what is transferred to the analyst is infantile urge; the past is reconstructed and old conflicts can be understood and resolved. But, due to the way in which this theory has been formulated, and because of their (natural) concern to avoid undue focus on past, rather than present and future, issues, existentialists remain wary of the concept.

Assuming that—to continue to use Freudian terminology—certain factors in the personality can be rendered unconscious (repressed) in a way that is harmful to the person, what are these factors? It is here, I think, that the main disagreement lies. Freud considered them to be derived from libidinal and aggressive instinctual urges. The Existential would, I assume, regard them as representations of the authentic self, although preferring the term 'alienation' to 'repression.' However, if it is recognized, by both schools of thought, that what is transferred to the analyst are primarily those urges of the self that have been denied expression, and that the authentic self is concerned not merely with past frustrations but with present and future possibilities of relationship, there would appear to be no inevitable reason for disagreement over this question.

The 'True' and the 'False' Self

The artist may be famed for the actual piece of work that he does, but the scientist who seeks distinction must discover a new thing or conceive a new law. In the field of psychoanalysis, where there is no firmly established language except that of Freud in which to describe the phenomena, those workers with personal ambition fall into the temptation of providing new verbal formulations, and this is perhaps one of the reasons for the existence of a superfluity of verbal concepts. It is important, therefore, to view any new terminology with circumspection. However, the distinction between the true (real) and the false self has two important merits: it is immediately meaningful in terms of human experience and it has arisen independently in the minds of several thinkers. But is it a distinction which will really enrich our theory of personality? Does it describe anything which the traditional psychoanalytic theory cannot?

Much, in fact, that is denoted by the word 'false' can be adequately accounted for by Freud's term, 'defensive.' A 'defence' is a manoeuvre to prevent the expression of an 'instinctual' impulse considered likely, for one reason or another, to have undesirable effects in life. The impulse in question will then be repressed (or suffer some other vicissitude such as projection), with the consequence that actual behaviour will no longer be a relatively accurate expression of personality but will give a false, disguised and distorted picture of it. A person who, for instance, has repressed viciousness may present a mild and equable demeanour. In terms of the dichotomy under consideration his 'instinctive' self is the true one, his defences and their consequences false. But suppose that his viciousness is not primary but is itself merely a disguise or a relatively meaningless escape valve? Does not one again have to put the question: 'Is his behaviour true or false?' And does not the Freudian theory become at this point—to say the least—unnecessarily complicated? Why did not Freud formulate his ideas in terms of trueness or authenticity? Chiefly, it would seem, because he used the biological framework. But there is, perhaps, another reason.

Freud's theory of human growth appears to be one of continuity: he has spelled out the ways in which the child is father to the man, the degree to which we carry our childhood with us; and, indeed, is often criticised for dwelling too much on ontological development. Yet he regarded growth less as a continuing evolution than as a gradual victory of each stage over the past; the 'pleasure principle' must succumb to the 'reality principle'; each new self discards the old, even if traces of it remain to harass and embarrass. Freud is here caught between the authenticity of the past and of the present, and his thinking does not allow for the unfolding of a true self which remains intact as the core of personality, a unique entity gathering meaning as it grows, discarding only those aims and illusions that are peripheral to its being, whose quality is measured not by stage of development, degree of libidinization, or physical mode of expression, but by its experienced meaningfulness and manifest spontaneity. In a theory of continuity the main dichotomy is not between the past and present or id and ego but between what is true and what is false.

Is it possible to reformulate Freud's theory—which can account, so nearly adequately, for so much—in these sort of terms without losing more than is gained?

A first move would seem to be the acceptance of Fairbairn's view that the infant state dissociates only in the face of adverse circumstances, and to equate this state with that of the true self, which is spontaneous, concerned with meaning and the agent of its own action. The integration is primary but not absolute, in that certain determinants of behaviour—such as reflex actions—have their own relative independence. These elements constitute behaviour which in animal life is called 'instinctual,' but it does not follow that the spontaneous urge of the true self lacks biological foundation.

In the imperfect world in which the true self finds itself it inevitably becomes modified in a way that fails to do justice to its potential. At what point does the distortion of the original urge become so marked as to justify the view that a 'false self' is operating? The answer to this would appear to be somewhat arbitrary, depending on whether one is an idealist or a cynic, and is equivalent to the vexed question which occurs in traditional psychoanalytical thought: 'When is behaviour "adaptive" and when "defensive"?' But it would perhaps be least confusing to restrict the term 'false' to behaviour designed, for whatever reason, to conceal the existence of the true self and therefore to deny meaning. The reasons for this kind of aim would include the avoidance of a real experience of life that was too awful to contemplate, the preservation (as Winnicott has shown) of a hidden but intact true self, and the attainment of some kind of meaning and satisfaction from the spurious personality which is erected. Although some satisfaction may be gained in this way, true meaning cannot. In such a state the person is 'depersonalized'; his identity is based on delusion and parasitism, dependent on the use of mechanisms known to psychoanalysts by such terms as introjection, identification, narcissism, masochism, and so on; he has become a quisling, and has, in Anna Freud's phrase, 'identified with the aggressor,' the latter being, in this context, the world which has prevented him from becoming himself. This kind of aim includes, but is much more extensive than, that covered by Freud's conception of the 'secondary gain of illness.'

Actual behaviour will necessarily be a function of both the true and the false. The person who has—if only temporarily—abandoned his main spontaneous urge to live will attempt to express it in whatever manner, however limited, that remains open to him. In his restricted state he may, if fortunate, find surprising yet creative ways of revealing his true self, as in the symbolism of art, but it is likelier—because easier—that he will be more able to give vent to, in distorted form, the destructive aspects of his real response to experience.

Any alteration in basic theoretical orientation will have an effect on clinical practice and on the way in which particular clinical states are formulated. What difference would be made by the change in emphasis under discussion? One might expect, for instance, that a psychoanalyst thinking in this kind of framework would focus on the authenticity of a piece of behaviour; that, for instance, he would be quick to consider whether the aggression of a paranoid patient was an attempt to ward off engulfment (being an expression of the true self) or was a pretence of aggression in order to give the impression that no such fear existed. Psychoanalysts do, of course, seek out such distinctions, but their present theoretical framework does not readily give them the mental set for such a task.

Hysteria

The division into true and false has so far been used in this essay, in considering schizoid states. Can it be applied to other clinical conditions? Let us take hysteria as an example.

According to current psychoanalytic theory, hysterical symptoms occur when an instinctive (usually sexual) urge is repressed and appears in symbolic form in an unexpected area of experience. For instance, a woman may repress a sexual impulse only to find herself plagued by a disturbance of swallowing; analysis reveals that, unconsciously, vaginal sensations have been displaced on to the mouth and pharynx. This kind of event (though usually in a much more complicated form than the example given) has frequently been described in the psychoanalytic literature, but is it sufficient to account for the main characteristic of hysteria: dramatization? It is a fact that the hysteric is acting a part in a play which exists in the realm of unconscious fantasy, but so are many people who lack the distinctive excitability and flair of the hysteric. Classical theory attempts to deal with this by the concept of 'hysterical character': whole areas of experience are 'libidinized,' giving an orgastic quality to behaviour. But this in turn is unsatisfactory. The behaviour in question is not merely orgastic (and it is not usually resolved by giving it this interpretation) but has a quality of pseudo-liveliness about it, as though the woman were trying to convince herself and others that she is alive, and very much so. And such a woman may well be having perfectly good orgasms all the time; the important question is whether her sexuality—and her behaviour in general—is true or false.

The idea that the dramatization of hysteria derives from a false self would seem to account for it more easily and more adequately than does the present theory. One is reminded of the little girl described by Winnicott who was gay and who danced beautifully to offset her mother's depression, and of the patients described by Melanie Klein as manifesting a 'manic defence' against depression. (There is a greater similarity between mania and hysteria than is easily accounted for.) The hysteric who so pitifully tries to present herself as real, lively, and desirable does so, perhaps, because her true self has been repressed; she feels an empty shell, yet those around expect vitality. An important differentiating factor in the aetiology of the false self of the schizoid and that of the hysteric may lie in the kind of personality demanded by the family into which he or she is born.

Inasmuch, then, as hysterical behaviour is false, the current psychodynamic theory is called into question, for the symptoms are less a distorted expression of the primary drive than a meaningless substitute for it. Freud has described the way in which a drive and its defence can be skilfully woven into a compromise symptom, and the primary drive no doubt reveals itself, when possible, even in the spurious activities of the hysteric; but it is likely that the real feelings which emerge are mainly aggressive ones and that much at present considered true (even if distorted) is really false. This would account for the fact that hysteria is a much more difficult condition to treat than would be expected if Freud's theory of it were quite correct. That sexuality plays such a central role in the condition may be due not merely to the fact that sexuality is one of the things which are repressed but that it is a suitable and powerful symbol of liveliness; and women may suffer from the disease more frequently than men because they get more encouragement, in our culture, to be false to themselves.

Psychic Economy

Although Freud understood his patients by discovering the meaning of their symptoms, his theory of personality is based on psychic economy—the distribution of energy within the mind. If one is to consider the possibility of developing a theory of mind based on the consequences of meaningful action where, if at all, does psychic economy play a part?

Even when discussing healthy, spontaneous behaviour we cannot, in fact, entirely disregard the question of psychic energy, for it is bound to influence our choice of action. I may wish to finish this essay at one sitting but I know that eventually, through mental fatigue, I would either have to stop or else severely limit my goal; and I think this would be true at a certain point even in the absence of neurotic inhibition.

In pathological states, however, psychic economy may restrict choice much more ruthlessly and perhaps even dictate the scene. So much energy may be lost through repression and dissociation or locked in the vicious circles of obsessional thinking that there is little left for the ordinary task of living. Moreover, the available energy may be of a different quality from the natural one, or forced to operate in a different way. When dissociation occurs—as it does in all mental ill-health— it is likely that energy takes on a cruder form; in the same way, perhaps, that there is a release of crude neuronal discharge from the brain stem when the cortex is put out of action. This could account, at least in part, for some of the clinical states associated with 'primitive' behaviour: urgency, impatience, anxiety, greed, rigidity, and so on.

A distinction of this kind between refined (integrated) and crude (disintegrated) energy brings to mind Freud's differentiation between the 'unbound' energy of the 'id' and the 'bound' energy of the 'ego.' Are they equivalent? In considering unbound energy to be primitive, Freud believed that it partook of the nature of the child, and it is possible that he was somewhat mistaken in this, underestimating the child's degree of integration and capacity for personal experience. (That he was—at least to a degree—is suggested by the work of Schachtel on infant development and by Rycroft on the activity of the 'id' and the 'ego.') If this is so, Freud is attributing a kind of normality (even if regressed) to this crude activity which it does not really possess, with the consequence that he may have seen meaning in it which is not there.

This line of thought has led to a paradoxical idea: that Freud, who (as I indicated at the beginning of this essay) seems to need to be defended against the accusation that his approach is too mechanistic, now appears to see meaning where he should be seeing mechanism (i.e., the inevitable consequences of psychic dissociation which are quite outside the scope of the person's will). If he has done this, then psychoanalysts have followed him—and gone further. Very few clinical psychoanalytic studies—Federn[12] being a brilliant exception—take much account of psychic economy. Melanie Klein, for instance, writes as though the correct therapeutic response to every psychopathological state is an interpretation, thereby assuming that the only bar to healthy functioning is a defensive strategy.

Because the great contribution of psychoanalysis has been to understand the meaning of symptoms, the fact that they may have overestimated the territory in which this is possible is perhaps inevitable and of secondary importance. But the error needs to be recognized for the sake of theory and practice. To know when a patient is so trapped by his psychic economy that he cannot, however willing, respond to interpretations, may be crucial, and a mistake of this kind is so painful to the patient that he may not easily forgive the analyst for making it. It is perhaps here that Winnicott's concept of 'holding,' rather than interpreting, the patient in certain critical states of mind is appropriate.

Another reason for mistakenly attributing meaning to a symptom is the natural fear which the psychoanalyst has of colluding with the patient's passive urge to renounce responsibility for his actions, an urge that is so widespread in our culture that Szasz[13] considers it to be the key to mental illness. Szasz is stimulating and in many ways convincing on this subject but it would seem that, by ignoring psychic economy, he overstates a valid and valuable case and may, like Melanie Klein, expect more from interpretations than is always possible.

Schizophrenia and the Family

In their recent book Sanity, Madness and the Family[14]—the first volume of a series—Laing and Esterson describe a study of families, one of whose members had been diagnosed by psychiatrists as schizophrenic. A notable feature of the recorded interviews is that little interpretation was made and the family was permitted to reveal itself with a minimum of interference.

Contrary to the expectations of current psychiatric thought, the authors found that the 'patient' presented a view of events, which, in their estimation, was often nearer the truth than that of the rest of the family. When she (the study was confined to female schizophrenics) revealed 'delusions' of persecution she was describing, in unusual and picturesque language, what was actually being done to her by the family at a certain level of experience. Her identity was being crushed because the family colluded, in cruel and subtle ways, in invalidating her experience of life, causing her to doubt the evidence of her senses. We are made to feel how, if we had been put in the same position as the 'victim,' we would have been hard pressed to find a better solution than she did.

These findings suggest to the authors that schizophrenia is not, as is commonly thought, a disease process, but the label attached to a certain type of behaviour shown by certain people who, having been subjected to strange experiences by their families, come, understandably, to behave in a strange way themselves. If this finding is correct—and the book is, by and large, convincing—it constitutes a very powerful opposition to the traditional psychiatric theory of the origin of schizophrenia, and, by demonstrating that pathogenic influences are being exerted by the family in the present, it challenges the psychoanalytic theory that schizophrenia originates in a faulty mother-infant set up. Recently David Cooper[15] has described an experimental approach to the organisation of a mental hospital ward based on ideas similar to those presented by Laing and Esterson.

This approach to schizophrenic families is not exclusive to the British Existentialist school of thought, for the most creative work in this area has been done earlier in America by Bateson and others, but it would seem that their conception of personality has helped the authors to explore very fruitfully the schizophrenic's search for identity and the truth in his apparently mad perceptions. One criticism which a psychoanalyst would make of their formulations, however favourable he might be to the work, is that the events are being described as though the 'patient' were contributing nothing to the disaster. The psychoanalysis of schizophrenia has shown that the pathological distortions of love and hate characteristic of this illness, engendered by whatever original causes, are self-destructive and involve a masochistic manipulation of others to behave badly towards the self. It is difficult to believe that this tendency does not contribute in some measure to the clinical picture described by Laing and Esterson, and a more likely assumption to make is that an early parent-child failure has been followed by a vicious circle in which both family and victim play their unhappy parts.

If this is correct, then the authors have shown a bias in which aggressive action is attributed to the parents (and siblings) alone. In one sense this is natural enough, for the authors are coming to the aid of someone whose voice has been unheard for too long. But perhaps there is more to it than this. Theoretical preoccupations tend to make workers selective in their perception of clinical phenomena, and in concentrating on the reality concealed in the patient's perception of others they may have overlooked some indirect methods of action used by him to express his identity. There is a possibility that the existentialists, although usefully emphasizing the agency of the person, may—paradoxically—by denying the validity of what psychoanalysts refer to as 'unconscious motivation' or 'repressed drive,' fail to see the agency of the person in certain pathological techniques.

Personal Relationships

In spite of the fact that he revealed much about human relationships, Freud was more concerned with intrapsychic phenomena and his theory reflected this preoccupation; nor has psychoanalysis been successful hitherto in finding a framework within which to describe what actually occurs between persons. This is a field in which one would expect the existentialists, who are concerned with 'Being-in-the-world' to have made some advance. How successful have they been?

In his article, 'Two Types of Rationality,'[16] David Cooper criticizes 'analytical rationality'—the traditional logic of human relationships in which truth is considered to lie outside the reality of the relationship, the observer and observed being in passive relationship with each other. By contrast:

> Human reality is that sector of reality where totalization is the very mode of being. A totality is something completed which therefore can be grasped as a whole; a totalization, on the other hand, is a perceptual movement ... What goes on in the reciprocal relation of a two-person transaction is as follows: I totalize you, but you, in your reciprocal totalization of me, include my totalization of you, so that my totalization of you involves a totalization of your totalization of me, and so on ....
>
> This view of human relations was anticipated by Sartre in his earlier work, *Being and Nothingness*, in a familiar example:
> I am surreptitiously looking through a keyhole at a scene in the next room. I become aware of a presence behind me. I turn and discover that someone has been watching me. At that moment a 'haemorrhage' occurs. The pure subjectivity that I have been existing as an observer of the scene in the next room drains away from my world into the world of the other where I become nothing more than a shameful object observed by him. At least until I find a way to regain my existence, return to the centre of my world and reduce the other in turn to being an object for me.[17]

This little example is evidently intended to convey what is typical of human relationships in general, yet the impression actually given is of a particular kind of relationship, one in which the two people are either unknown to each other, or, if known, do not possess a sense of mutual trust and affection. There is an assumption that the first person (at the keyhole) deeply minds the unexpected observation of the second, will necessarily cringe before his glance, and that his only mode of recovering his sense of dignity and identity is by retaliatory observation. There would appear to be no possibility, in this formulation of the scene, that a relationship might exist between the two people that is characterized by love and which transcends or precludes the shame and disintegration. Or that, if shame occurs, that it might be followed by acceptance and growth rather than retaliation. (I do not mean to imply that I believe in the existence of relationships so ideal that the participants do not sometimes act in a retaliatory way upon each other, but that it is a mistake to assume it to be the natural, inevitable reaction.)

The type of relationship formulated by Cooper would seem to be one in which elements of control, manipulation, and narcissistic assertion are uppermost; the conception of an atmosphere of love, trust, defencelessness, contemplation is lacking. Once again there is a paradox. The psychology that is attempting to describe the possibilities of human freedom finds itself not necessarily more successful in the attempt than those before it.

In *The Self and Others*[17] Laing uses the terminology of 'person perception psychology,' a phenomenological approach, developed by Heider and others, to describe human relationships, in which the implicit attributions people make about each other are carefully analyzed. The usefulness of this language, however, remains in doubt; it shows signs of becoming lost in mathematical formulae, a fate which befell the promising work of Kurt Lewin.

Laing is a perceptive clinician and a vigorous and creative thinker who makes use of whatever bits of language he can lay his hands on, and for this reason *The Self and Others* is a rewarding book. It does not follow from this that the terminology of 'person perception psychology' is entirely safe as a basis for a study of relationships. There is a dilemma in that all descriptions of human behaviour that depart from ordinary language are in danger of leading us into the very kind of arid, atomistic, mechanistic world which the Existentialists are so anxious to avoid. The need for a satisfactory language with which to discuss relationships in a scientific way is a pressing one and has not yet been met.

Existentialism and Psychoanalysis

Existentialism has a theoretical orientation more suited to the study of persons than has that of psychoanalysis. In this country its exponents are characterized by a preoccupation with schizophrenia, a tendency to support the underdog, a leaning towards the philosophy of Sartre—and courage—and have already made some useful contributions to an understanding of schizoid states and, especially, of the relationships within a family containing a schizophrenic member.

The potential of this new approach is limited, at present, by the fact that some fruitful channels opened by psychoanalysis are being neglected. Can the existentialists afford to put aside the technique of 'transference' interpretation? To what degree does their work suffer if they do not take into consideration the two types of symbolic thinking described by Freud as 'primary process' (typified by dreams) and 'secondary process' (typified by conscious logic)? Have they paid sufficient attention to guilt, mourning and depression, to psychic economy, to child development, or to the fact that there are two sexes involved in human intercourse?

Psychotherapy constitutes the only real challenge and alternative to the organic school of psychiatry that holds sway in our country, and its practitioners cannot afford to be catastrophically divided among themselves. It would be a great pity if the Freudian and Existential schools of thought grew apart rather than together.

References

1. Jones, Ernest (1953), *Sigmund Freud, vol. 1: Life and Work*, Basic Books, New York.
2. Freud, Sigmund (1955), *The Interpretation of Dreams*, Basic Books, New York.
3. Home, H. J. (1966), 'The Concept of Mind,' *Int. J. Psychoanal.* 47, pp. 42–49.
4. Hartmann, Heinz (1964), *Essays on Ego Psychology*, International Universities Press, New York.
5. Erikson, E. H. (1959), 'Identity and the Life Cycle,' *Psychol. Issues* 1, 1.
6. May, Rollo et al., eds. (1958), *Existence*, Basic Books, New York.
7. Laing, R. D. (1965), *The Divided Self*, Penguin Books, New York.
8. Maxwell, Gavin (1965), *The House of Elrig*, Dutton, New York.
9. Klein, Melanie (1948), *Contributions to Psychoanalysis*, 1921–1945, Hillary House, New York; (1932), *The Psychoanalysis of Children*, 3d ed., Hillary House, New York; Melanie Kliein et al. (1936), *Developments in Psychoanalysis*, Hillary House, New York.
10. Winnicott, D. W. (1957), 'Reparation in Respect of Mother's Organised Defence against Depression,' in *Collected Papers*, Basic Books, New York.
11. Sartre, J. P. (1964), *Being and Nothingness*, translated by H. E. Barnes, Citadel, New York.
12. Federn, Paul (1953), *Ego Psychology and the Psychoses*, Basic Books, New York.
13. Szasz, Thomas S. (1961), *The Myth of Mental Illness*, Harper, New York.
14. Laing, R.D. and A. Esterson (1965), *Sanity, Madness and Family, vol. 1: Families of Schizophrenics*, Basic Books, New York.
15. Cooper, David (1965), 'The Anti-Hospital: An Experiment in Psychiatry,' *New Society* (11 March) 5, p. 128.
16. Cooper, David (1965), 'Two Types of Rationality,' *New Left Review* (Jan-Feb), no. 29, pp. 62–68.
17. Laing, R.D. (1961), *The Self and Others*, Tavistock, London.

16

On Setting up a Psychotherapy Training Scheme

> *The more systematically education is planned, the more it is a matter of accident or luck whether education as initiation into conscious living still takes place at all.*
> —Peter Sloterdijk

In the last two decades several thinkers and researchers have shown the ways in which educational institutions constrain the discourse that takes place within them, thus preventing creative growth. In might be thought that psychotherapy, an undertaking designed to give maximum freedom to self-expression, would be an exception, but unhappily this is not always the case. For this reason a number of us in Cambridge felt the need to find a different approach to learning, avoiding the tendency to rigid hierarchy, discussions conducted in jargon incomprehensible to the ordinary citizen. While valuing the work of Freud and other major thinkers, we deplored the tendency to regard them as sacred texts from which deviations should be viewed with alarm or seem as manifestations of psychopathology. It the light of these ideas it seemed a worthwhile undertaking to set up a teaching scheme in which people could learn the practice of psychotherapy in an atmosphere as free as possible from these limitations.

This chapter emerged from talks between the author, Lucy King and Carol Naughton, and the penultimate draft was discussed with the training group as a whole.

The present climate of opinion in Britain is unfavourable to such endeavours. Permissiveness—whether in school or university—tends to be regarded as an idealistic dream of the 1960s and, by contrast, there is a return to authoritarian teaching methods and an increased focus on training for jobs. The contemporary distrust of liberal ideals has led to a certain amount of caution.

The Cambridge Psychotherapy Training Group

The group began in 1980 when a small number of people came together in Cambridge with the aim of providing a learning environment for those who wished to become psychotherapists. Some of this group were trained therapists, some potential students. Our aim was not to organise a training course in psychotherapy similar to those existing elsewhere but to explore the possibilities of learning therapy according to a certain ideology. We centred on the belief that the most profitable way to learn psychotherapy is in a setting in which students have as much autonomy as can be managed and can develop their own approach in their own way and their own time rather than having a structured course imposed on them. The training we offer can therefore be seen to mirror the experience of being in a therapy which emphasis mutuality; and it is supported by our belief that only in a free, open dialogue can genuine learning and creative exploration take place. The group, therefore, is not organised in a conventionally hierarchical way. It has no explicit power structure. There is no chairman or training committee. Decisions are made by the group as a whole. There are no rules as such. Although one of the students acts as a secretary and there is a small administrative group, there is no formal committee or written regulation. It is, however, expected that students will have personal therapy and supervision and that before they finish training they will have had an appropriate variety and depth of practical experience as therapists. But we do not specify lengths of time for these undertakings.

None the less we seek to be informal, to be worthy of (self-) respect without compromising our integrity in the pursuit of conventional respectability. Our dilemmas over this are exemplified by the naming of the group. We have a formal, name-on-notepaper: The Cambridge Psychotherapy Training Group. More commonly we are known as the Outfit. Originally coined, somewhat jokingly, as an in-house anti-name, this has now escaped into more general usage. Meetings are held at each other's houses. In order to preserve as much spontaneity as possible and to allow for ideas and interests to be pursued as they arise we have no set, yearly curriculum and the planning of meetings ahead is of a limited nature.

However much we attempt to avoid a gap between students and therapists, it is recognised that their needs are different. The students are undertaking to turn themselves into therapists; they want a career. For this reason they are prepared to put more time and energy into the project. The role of the therapists is more ambiguous.

Theoretical Orientation

All of the therapists who have joined the group have a particular, albeit broad, theoretical orientation. Although not adherents to any specific school of thought (e.g., Freudian, Jungian) their approach could be called, for want of a better term, that of psychoanalytically orientated psychotherapy—provided that this does not imply a watered down version of psychoanalysis and allows for the fact that we aim to explore the boundaries of contemporary theory and practice. Students are not only introduced to analytical concepts (transference, countertransference, and so on) but offered the means to make a critique of these concepts. One focus of interest has gradually emerged. Those who have been attracted to a group which attempts to minimise hierarchical power have shown a characteristic attitude to the way in which psychotherapy is conducted. In discussion, the concealed power that often lies behind interpretations and other interventions is consistently challenged, and ways are sought of avoiding unnecessary inequality in therapy and formulating theories to match this endeavour. It seems likely that this focus on the question of power in the therapeutic relationship will continue to colour our orientation and may prove to be the growing point of our ideas.

Even though an organisation may have an ethos and structure aimed at achieving equality of power—as does the Outfit—there are likely to be factors which cause certain individuals or sub-groups to have undue influence. Age, experience, and personal assertiveness will inevitably play their part. In the case of a group which is still in the early stages of development there is an additional factor. When someone, or a small number of people, initiate a new training scheme they are bound to have an emotional stake in its remaining basically true to the early ideas. Regarded positively this can be seen as an important creative vision without which the organisation would not have come to exist and a telling factor in preserving new thinking in the face of pressure to conform to conventional styles. But there are also dangers in this; the originators may become too protective of the vision and too possessive of the group. (The situation is, of course, more complex, for those who join later are not necessarily more orthodox in their thinking or less passionate in their identification with the aims of the project.) The group has, in any event, found it necessary to engage with this kind of problem.

The emotional dilemma between therapists and their students/patients who meet each other in the ordinary course of teaching is always a major problem in any psychotherapeutic training scheme. When the set-up is small, informal, and situated in a city of modest size with relatively few experienced therapists this predicament can be extreme, leading to tensions and inhibitions, many of which are covert. One student felt such discomfort when his therapist was present in the group that he left to train elsewhere. (This did not, however, appear to affect his therapy adversely and he rejoined the group after his training finished.) In a more formal organisation there would be less contact between students and therapists, probably less self-revelation and less likelihood of open embarrassment and conflict. Whatever the structure of the group tensions between the student and therapist cannot be avoided. It is, of course, well known that the transference problems which attend any training analysis are formidable.[1] We have no evidence that they are more difficult in this kind of group than in a hierarchical one. Indeed, the lack of hierarchy and the fact that the therapists have no formal power over the students and no influence in assessing their progress to qualify may lessen the likelihood of a persistent transference. If this were the case it would be in keeping with my view, argued elsewhere,[2] that the more a sense of equality can be experienced between the therapist and patient the less likely is an idealised transference to reach unmanageable and unnecessary dimensions.

The Style of the Discussions

Many of the early discussions tackled questions about the nature, morality, and political and religious meanings of psychotherapy. From

On Setting up a Psychotherapy Training Scheme 241

the beginning we have attempted to bring as fresh and unbiased an approach to the study of psychotherapy as we can muster, encouraging participants to draw from their own life-experience as well as from the practise of therapy and the reading of books. This not only enabled beginners to participate more easily but was a recognition that their 'naïve' contributions often proved stimulating and productive. It was an emphasis, however, which led to our first major confrontation with each other. The problem was as follows:

1. As the group increased in size and as more trained therapists joined us, the discussions became a less satisfactory forum for the expression of tentative, untutored, and personal exploration, and conversations became dominated, at the expense of the students, by those members of the group who had more clinical experience, more confidence, and more familiarity with psychoanalytic terminology. The students themselves were divided on this issue. While some felt that they gained knowledge by listening to the therapists discussing their work and ideas, others experienced great frustration in losing the opportunity to explore their own ideas in a way that had previously been possible. When this dilemma was brought into the open a further problem developed. Some of the therapists then felt inhibited in their own self-expression. How could they bring zest and creativity into the discussions in a way that fulfilled their personal needs and enabled them to make a valuable contribution if they were to be stifled? This seemed particularly hard since the therapists are not paid: they are here, presumably, to enjoy themselves, gain illumination, and have the satisfaction of acting as facilitators for students to learn to be therapists.

2. There were disagreements about the relative merits of unstructured discussions and organised meetings in which topics were planned beforehand according to a curriculum. Some members felt that without planning of this kind, and perhaps lacking a more formal teaching set-up, important subjects would be omitted and the course would not constitute a proper training—or would not be seen to do so.

The fact that these difficulties have been aired appears to have gone some way towards alleviating them. Nevertheless meetings of the Outfit as a whole lack the ease and bonhomie of the student group and we need to explore the matter further. One practical measure we have taken is to reduce their frequency, and they now occur once a month. It is noticeable that when we arrange to have a speaker, the focus thus provided seems to facilitate discussions between therapists and students. The students meet once a week or more and are sometimes joined by one or two of the therapists. With this kind of distribution of experience the discussions usually go well. These changes have, by and large, been initiated by the students. As a consequence the student group has become more coherent; members are more confident, have a greater sense of direction, and enjoy themselves more.

The Students' Work

Students learn at their own pace and establish their priorities at each point of their training in relation to personal therapy, supervision, theory, and practical (therapeutic) work. For some students one of these aspects of training may be uppermost; for others, integration of the different forms of learning may be paramount. As the teaching is not organised according to a routine pattern new students take their time in getting the feel of this kind of training. It was decided not to establish a set reading list however helpful and comforting such a list might be. Topics and related reading are now organised in advance. The length of time spent on any topic is decided by the student group as a whole at the beginning of the study period.

In the interests of mutual understanding and teaching, students have set up smaller groups—mainly pairs—in which papers and books are read together, work with patients is discussed and ideas, doubts, and confusions are shared. The pairings are changed every six months, giving students a chance to get to know each other's work throughout the years of training. It is a mode of learning which requires a great deal of maturity and dedication from students. Fortunately they are helped by the fact that Cambridge has a wealth of psychotherapeutic lectures and discussions of high calibre, most of which they can attend.

The Therapists

Because the students are responsible for their own training, the position of therapists is much less clear than is usually the case in comparable organisations. That the experience and support of the therapist is valued by the students is unquestionable, but their sense of identity is vulnerable, their formal role continues to be under discussion and they have difficulty in establishing themselves as a coherent and purposeful group in the way that the students have done. Their function is perhaps best described as that of a resource network—members offer the kind of help each of them individually feels best at giving, and (not least importantly) engage in those activities that they enjoy and find stimulating. They participate in discussions, sometimes as leaders or facilitators and they make themselves available to students to discuss all aspects of training, both individual and group. They are not paid for any of their work except when a student chooses to make a contract for individual therapy or supervision with an Outfit therapist.

The therapists meet from time to time to discuss theory, practice, and any matters of mutual interest including their function in the Outfit. We feel that, amongst other things, the group provides a useful transitional forum for those students who have recently qualified.

Selection

One of the very few formal procedures we have adopted is that of admitting new students. They are invited to meet, individually, a few members of the group, and if this goes well they join one of the meetings before a decision is made. The interviews are structured, as far as possible, on the basis of equality, that is to say, the applicants are encouraged to scrutinise us as thoroughly as we scrutinise them. There are no formal criteria for acceptance by us. We are looking for people whose commitment to becoming a therapist is strong, who appear to have the necessary sensitivity for the work, and who, by virtue of their worldview, are likely to feel at home in a group of this kind.

It is the last of these criteria which has made selection an arduous and time-consuming task. In particular, the fact that students need to be able to teach each other means we must try to select those applicants who will be receptive to the needs of the group and its individual members.

Graduation

One of our aims is to provide the kind of setting that will best enable a student to gain realistic evidence of her or his progress during the course of training. When, however, we come to the final evaluation of the student's overall capability, problems arise. In our view the conventional methods of assessment at the end of training are unsatisfactory, and the results of such measures unimpressive. The correlation between successful qualification and actual therapeutic ability is, to put it mildly, not as close as one might hope for. Moreover, the disadvantages of such methods are many: the criteria are selective and stifle creativity of thought; the values tend to be based on respectability and prestige; the criteria used are often quantitative (how many patients seen, and so forth) and are a poor substitute for really knowing the students and their work. Most of all, we wish to avoid having a group in which evaluation is emphasised at the expense of creative and lively interchange.

With these thoughts in mind we place emphasis on self-responsibility and openness in personal communication in the hope that it will thereby be unlikely for a totally unsuitable student to stay with us for a period of years and that in most cases student and group will be able to gauge a time when enough training has been accomplished.

If the group is prepared to say with integrity that a certain student has been accepted as a trained member it would seem necessary to reserve the right to refuse such an endorsement. However, from our experience hitherto, we believe that to do so would be a drastic and *exceptional* move. A custom has emerged whereby students present themselves to the group when they feel ready to do so. There is no formula for this presentation and students have their own individual ways of conveying their attitudes, beliefs, and the nature of their practice. A further custom is that students who become accepted as trained therapists mark the occasion by a ritual or celebration of their choice.

There is always a balance to be made between the practical needs of a group and its ideals. In the present economic and moral climate it is difficult to justify, and put into practice, a teaching scheme with radical aims. Our best hope lies in the fact that the Outfit shows no sign of becoming ossified; it has remained sufficiently flexible for us to continue to make changes without threatening the whole edifice, and the enthusiasm with which students work together to form a coherent training program increases each year.

We are currently negotiating for membership of the United Kingdom Standing Conference on Psychotherapy. It may be that in order to maintain our integrity we shall have to present our work in an individual way rather than one which conforms to the conventionally accepted manner of doing so. The validity of our endeavour depends, in the end, on the quality of the group—its openness, spontaneity, goodwill, rigour, and firmness.

The following brief description of the experience of training was written by two students nearing graduation:

> We began the training as two quite different people and have both been changed by the experience. However, we do not feel we have been cloned in that process. We emerge with our individuality intact.
>
> To begin with there was a necessary period of establishing personal therapy, settling into the group and developing a sense of membership. The student and large-group meetings which have been described earlier in the chapter provided the central opportunities for discussion of theoretical, philosophical, practical, and organisational issues.
>
> We have particularly valued the unstructured meetings which take place occasionally in the student group when time is made available for more spontaneous discussion, offering an opportunity for all students to contribute from their life-experience. Other important aspects of the training have been small reading groups and regular meetings in pairs for shared learning of various kinds. We have both read widely and eclectically from the psychodynamic literature according to personal and group inclination and have also looked to novels, poetry, and drama for some of our stimulation.
>
> Our individual therapy has formed an integral part of the training, as it does elsewhere. When we felt ready to do so we began to see clients under supervision, beginning with one or two people and building a caseload slowly. We both have experience of more than one supervisor and of both individual and group supervision. We have also taken part in the process of interviewing and selecting new members, and are currently negotiating our graduation process in consultation with the rest of the group.
>
> There have, of course, been frustrations and negative experiences, especially over time spent on administration, sorting out differences of opinion and trying to reach agreement. There has been uncertainty and introspection about what are the essential elements of a good training in analytic psychotherapy. The group has sometimes seemed over-concerned with self-questioning, when perhaps the time could have been better spent getting on with the business of learning. These problems may arise both from the newness of the training and its unorthodoxy.
>
> It has been a problem that some personal issues which affect the dynamics of the student group cannot be dealt with, as they might be elsewhere, in an experiential group. We are a work group united by basic aims and a shared philosophy, and decisions have to be taken and actions agreed. Predictably tensions have developed in a gathering of independent and strong-minded individuals who expect to play their part in the development of their own learning.
>
> Another frustration that may have arisen from the group's unorthodoxy concerns the determination to avoid models of education that infantilize those who are students. In the Outfit this goes further than 'student-centred learning,' for we are not only concerned with learning and teaching but also with its underlying structures. Many training courses are lived through a metaphor of infancy-childhood-adoles-

cence. It is common at the beginning of such courses to experience oneself as 'the baby of the group,' later settling for a while into comfortable conformity, and then to experiment, rebel, and challenge. There are always staff members, hallowed texts or the institution itself to be loved, blamed, raged against, or relied upon.

The Outfit makes it difficult for students to sustain this metaphor. There is no institution, no training committee, no sacred text. The positive side of this is the possibility of adult relationships, mature responsibility, and real learning. On the negative side it may limit the possibility of useful dependency on more experienced people, increase uncertainties about the validity of the training, and create anxieties that are hard to bear.

This situation may also have contributed to some of the tensions and ambivalence between trained people and students over the role of the former. For example, we may want them as equals but can also sometimes experience them as neglectful parents. Although we free ourselves of the structures of the infantilizing institution we may still carry expectations and needs of it within us.

Other positive aspects of the training are that we have been free to learn at our own pace and have gained from participation in the personal and collective responsibility for the learning process among students and trained members. The emphasis on an understanding and challenging of power relationships, both in therapy and education, has been of central importance; as has the belief that, without sacrificing standards and rigour, a sensitive and responsive therapist can only be produced by a sensitive and responsive training.

These qualities and the explicit value placed on maturity gained in other areas of life have contributed to an experience which is unlike anything either of us has found in any other form of education or training. We have been part of a learning process which has provided us with a valid and valued experience which we could not easily have found elsewhere.

Rosemary Randall
Vivienne Seymour-Clark

Postscript 1997

A lot of water has flowed under the bridge in the last six years. An increase in size and, in particular, the difficulty of presenting ourselves as sufficiently 'normal' to be accepted for registration, have forced changes on us, some of which will be described in the next chapter. Nevertheless, the basic principles outlined here remain intact.

References

1. Roustang, F. (1976), *Dire Mastery*, translated by N. Lackacher, Johns Hopkins University Press, Baltimore, MD.
2. Lomas, P. (1978), *The Limits of Interpretation*, Penguin, Harmondsworth.

17

The Teaching of Psychotherapy

> *Unless we purposely turn our eyes to look at something that interests us as individuals, we shall literally see nothing in the world, and we shall understand nothing the in the real world unless we remember that we freely choose the direction in which to look.*
> —Stuart Hampshire

Our views on how psychotherapy is best learnt and taught are inevitably influenced by our philosophy of education in general. Do psychotherapists, as a group, have a particular line on this? One clue to a possible answer is the way in which psychotherapists try to influence their patients—that is to say, in what way they attempt to give a needed insight to another.

The tradition in which those of us work who have been strongly influenced by Freud is to place interpretation at the centre of our attempt to influence. In other words, we are not didactic. We do not say to the patient: 'This is what you must think; this is what you must believe.' We try, using our knowledge and privileged position, to understand what the patient wishes to convey to us of what is most profound in them, and inform them of our impression. It is, by and large, a permissive method, allowing the patient much freedom of expression. In practice, however, there is often less freedom than the

---

Originally read to The Severnside Society for Psychotherapy, Bristol, May 1993

theory suggests. Freud emphasised the prevalence of resistance to interpretation and the amount of determination and persistence necessary to overcome the patient's denials. In Freud's conception of psychoanalysis it is the practitioner who has the truth, who knows what the patient should learn, and who has a body of knowledge and theory at his disposal unavailable to the patient. The fact that Freud eschewed blatant didacticism like the plague and developed a method which gave the patient incomparably more freedom to express themselves than had hitherto been possible in psychiatry is a paradox which, I believe, inhibits our ability to see the one-sidedness of his conversations with patients. Nevertheless, in recent years, due to rigorous scrutiny of Freud's work, we are now in a better position to see the degree of coercion he imposed upon them. If we focus on this element in Freud's method (in particular, as it appears in some of his case-histories) it begins to look rather like a pedagogic form of education.

Since Freud formulated his ideas, the patient has increasingly come to be conceived by psychotherapy as a unique being capable of developing creatively if given the space to do so, as free as possible from the preoccupations and countertransference impediments of the therapist. In other words, there has been a shift, albeit a partial one, from the idea of a technique imposed on the patient towards the provision of what Winnicott refers to as a 'medium for growth' or 'facilitating environment.' This move, expressed so vividly by Winnicott, is also to be found in the work of several other thinkers, notably the Existential psychotherapists, and words and phrases, such as encouragement, holding, self-actualisation, person-centred therapy, empathy, and negative capability have become part of our professional language.

Although there is a wide variation in the exact stance which psychotherapists take on this issue, an increasing number of therapists—of whom I count myself one—are inclining to the view, present in Freud and now emerging more clearly, that the patient should be given respect as a being who is never completely knowable, cannot be fitted into any formula and needs to be encouraged to present his or her uniqueness; and that the therapist is more aptly considered as a midwife than a container of insights to pass on to the patient. We are, in a sense, becoming less confident.

If our theory of education in the consulting room has always been, and is increasing so, slanted towards the autonomy of the patient, how does this attitude stand in relation to theories of education in general?

The philosophy of education has, with a few exceptions, focused almost exclusively on the teaching of children, particularly small children. As far as I understand it as a non-expert, the seminal creative figures in the field—Rousseau, Pestalozzi, Froebel, Dewey, and Montessori—promote what is often called 'progressive education.' In his paper, 'Teaching and learning psychotherapy,' Michael Evans[1] describes this tradition as supporting 'the notion that the capacity to learn is inherent and that the function of education is to promote personal autonomy and creative capacities, and to enable knowledge to be regarded as a means of discovery.'
He quotes Dewey:

> To the growth of the child all studies are subservient; they are instruments valued as they serve the needs of growth. Personality, character, is more than subject matter. Not knowledge but self realisation is the goal. Moreover, subject matter never can be got into the child from without. Learning is active. It involves reaching out of the mind. It involves organic assimilation starting from within. The only significant method is the method of the mind as it reaches out and assimilates.[2]

In contrast to this philosophy Evans describes the traditional conventions of higher education.

> In Higher Education the prevailing method consists of the lecture or demonstration, closely followed by the seminar and the tutorial. At postgraduate level the tutorial takes precedence over the seminar and the lecture, and the student is expected to work more independently but is often isolated from other students because of his specialisation. These practices are characterised by an unquestioned common sense hierarchy, in which lecturers teach and students learn.
>
> The common assumption behind this system is that education consists of the transmission of culture by teachers which is received by pupils. At a later stage these facts and ideas are reproduced and it is assumed that learning has taken place. (Students frequently sell their books after their exams as if to demonstrate that their qualification proves that they have learned the contents.) The lecture theatre and even to some extent the seminar room are organised to express this hierarchy and the teachers exert their control and mastery through the system of devising aims and objectives, setting the syllabus, producing lecture lists, essay titles, marking systems, assessment criteria, and examinations.

In the fields of education, philosophy, and psychotherapy it has, in recent years, been suggested that the best way of reaching the truth is by conversation.* A conversation—a good conversation—is open-

---

* The Socratic dialogues precede this approach by two millennia, but Socrates was, in his subtle way, a very dominating teacher and perhaps not a good model in this context.

ended; there is no leader, no voice that is necessarily dominating, no truth other than the nearest approximation to it that will be arrived at by a group of people sufficiently relaxed and free from fear and constraint to say what they really think; and the due respect appropriate to those with much to contribute will not be allowed to inhibit the creative ideas of those whose knowledge of the matter under discussion is less at the moment; there are no prizes and no rewards other than enjoyment, play, curiosity and, if luck holds, some achievement.

Where, at the present time, does the teaching of psychotherapy stand in relation to the differing ideas on education? In some ways it stands clearly in the progressive tradition: the pupil gets more individual attention, by means of personal therapy and supervision, than perhaps in any other occupation. Moreover, this attention is centred on his or her uniqueness and the limitations that stand in the way of fruitful living; even in supervision, the student's individual responses (the countertransference) gains increasing emphasis. Also, as in progressive education, the focus is on activity: the student learns by doing: he or she sees clients.

In other ways, however, the progressive tendency is less in evidence and follows the conventions of traditional higher education: the transmission of culture by teachers which is received by pupils; teachers devise and organise a system of learning which students follow: there are assessment criteria and some kind of examination. To my mind this system is as inappropriate to the teaching of adults as of children and particularly inappropriate to the teaching of psychotherapy, a subject that depends far more on ordinary capacities of living (which teachers share with students and all members of the human race) than, for example, a much more technical undertaking like electronic engineering.

It was this line of thought that led some of us in Cambridge to set up a teaching scheme in psychotherapy, one in which the students' own drive to learn would constitute the energy by which the teaching scheme functioned and developed.* It was central to our thinking that students should be encouraged to learn and develop in their own unique way and their own time and expect to be able to turn to each other for help in learning. There were to be no fixed conditions or rules.

It is now clear to us that we were pursuing an aim which, however

---

* I write about the early days of this endeavor in chapter 16.

justifiable as a valid method, could not be maintained in the modern world. There is now a widespread belief that training set-ups should be regulated by a central body in order that the public be protected from morally irresponsible and ignorant practitioners, that such a central body could effectively bring this happy state about and that it could do so without stifling the expression of individuality in students and training organisations. This is a view which, I believe, involves a misunderstanding of the nature of good therapy and fails to recognise the gross distortions to creative work which such standardisations will bring. Nevertheless, in order to give our students a better chance of succeeding to achieve the necessary status to do the work they wanted to do we elected to follow the trend. However, within this limitation, we have tried to keep to our original aim as far as possible. There is no formal hierarchy. What students do is decided among themselves and there is no compulsion for individual students to follow any course of action with which they disagree. Nevertheless, certain expectations have developed which, although few, have a force comparable to rules, for example, that candidates should be prepared to have individual therapy and supervision for a substantial—though unspecified—period.

In practice what does this regime amount to? The students meet weekly to discuss psychotherapy; sometimes they invite one of the trained members to join them either as a participant in the discussion, or to lead a seminar, or give a talk; each month the whole group meets to discuss psychotherapy, sometimes inviting an outside speaker. The students arrange their own programme, usually planning meetings for a few months ahead, and, from time to time inviting one or two therapists to help them with their planning. It is understood that therapists are willing to meet any student to discuss a particular problem or advise on any matter, but this kind of help is, in fact, seldom asked for. Small study groups are arranged from time to time on an ad hoc basis. One of the problems is that, as therapists are not paid for the help they give, students are understandably reluctant to ask them to give their time. Occasionally the students have made a financial arrangement with a therapist to provide a weekly series of seminars over a period of time; but this is not the norm. The group functions, to some extent, as a network. This has been formalised by an arrangement of pairings lasting six months each, by means of which members meet each other informally to discuss psychotherapy or anything else they like, and to give each other mutual support. It is hard to overestimate the value students find in this arrangement.

I do not present this account as an ideal way of doing things, nor am I attempting to describe a group in which all is harmonious and we are on our way to heaven. It has, like any group, its own particular awfulness. But it is a different way of doing things and it appears to be able to foster the growth of therapists who show no obvious signs of being less competent or professionally dedicated than do other trainings in the field.

One of the difficulties of giving a description of a teaching scheme is that we are easily drawn towards specifying the organisation and the practical arrangements and leaving out of account the philosophy which informs the arrangements. The result is rather like that which follows from describing, in a mechanical way, the practicalities of psychotherapy—the setting, the cost, the frequency, and so on—without saying what it is all about and what it feels like to be doing it. Yet what really matters in what we do as a teaching group is to keep in mind the principles and aims which brought us together and to observe, for example, whether we do manage to create an atmosphere in which conversations of the kind I have mentioned can occur and what appear to be the advantages and disadvantages of so doing.

The reasons which make it difficult to maintain the ideals of a training of this kind, and which have revealed themselves in our own group, seem to fall into three categories:

1. *Practical.* As the group grows in size it grows in complexity. In order to facilitate communication, avoid muddle and save time, more organisation and division of labour becomes necessary. This is at the cost of flexibility and intimacy. For example, we now have business meetings with prearranged agendas and minutes which are basically no different from those in most organisations, and out of these meetings come fixed procedures. To put the matter another way, it becomes more difficult to rely on the kind of goodwill and personal understanding of each other that makes for congenial family life, and therefore procedures are established.

2. *Emotional.* A set-up that is not based on rules and in which structures are at a minimum requires its members—particularly those who are students—to tolerate a considerable level of uncertainty. Security has to be based on the member's own self-motivation and on personal trust in other members and less on a fixed framework and

procedure. The insecurity shows itself, I believe, in attempts to establish hierarchies which are not formalised and in attempts to control the activities of others and to discourage idiosyncracies. For this reason, the original idea that each student should be allowed as far as possible to learn, and to help others, in his or her own particular way is hard to maintain. It is, of course, quite realistic for the views of the more experienced therapists to be given due weight, but I believe that this is a different matter from the degree of control which can easily be exerted by the 'elders'—or indeed, by the organisation as a whole.

3. *The pull of cultural expectations.* Any organisation which departs radically from the normal way of doing things is under constant pressure from the outer world to get back into step and it does seem to be the case that the creative edge of most organisations gradually succumbs to this pressure. There is no doubt in my mind that the greatest obstacle to our endeavour has been, and will continue to be, the necessity to present ourselves in a way that is acceptable for a national Register. This has not only proved difficult in practice but has tested our capacity, consciously and unconsciously, to maintain confidence in our ideals in the face of obligations to conform to the generally accepted pattern. The pressure towards normalisation comes not only from outside but is in the individual members. Habit, as William James has so eloquently taught us, is a powerful force. And those of us who have worked in organisations in which the traditional hierarchies and procedures flourish tend to fall back on these methods when trying to solve problems. Moreover, members who are new to the group often find it difficult to believe that the flexibility which it promotes is really there. For example, students from time to time ask if a certain line of behaviour is 'permitted' rather than saying 'Do you think this would be a good thing to do?'

There is one particular area which proves to be a persistent problem: that of assessment and graduation. Appropriate, wise, and unbiased feedback from others is a vital element in learning. However, the word 'assessment' usually carries connotations of an examination in which the degree of overall competence of the student is the matter in question. In other words, help with creativity can easily become muddled with judgement of capacity. Thus a student may not be clear as to whether he or she is writing an essay for their personal development or in order to satisfy expectations or demands of others. To the degree that a student feels watched and judged by an organisation that is concerned with fitness to practice he or she will be insecure and less able to think boldly and creatively. Moreover, the time and energy absorbed by a preoccupation with assessment (which is part of the spirit of the age—we see it in schools, for example) could more effectively be used to help students in other ways.

Although there would be undoubted merits in having a means by which practitioners can be identified as having been well-trained these are not as unambiguously useful as might be supposed. The stamp of authority given by a qualification is, sadly, no guarantee that the practitioner is a good therapist, or a good therapist for a particular patient, and the apparent guarantee can inhibit the potential patient from finding an intuitive answer to the question 'Is this the right person to help me?' The criteria which one should use in estimating whether someone is capable of practising good therapy are elusive, for psychotherapy is, I believe, more akin to an art than a science and is probably best served by intimate experience of the student and our best intuitive judgment, rather than, say, the writing of a paper or a quantitative measure of training achieved. There is no satisfactory answer to this problem at present. But I believe that a shift from measures such as assessment, monitoring, and examination to the provision of a culture in which individual style, exploration, and self-responsibility are given as much rein as possible provides our best chance of helping prospective psychotherapists to be effective.

What we actually teach will vary according to our theoretical and ideological predilections, but I imagine that therapists influenced by Freud would give a lot of weight to his ideas on resistance, transference, and the influence of childhood experience. However, if there is merit in the view that psychotherapy is more akin to an art than a science, it follows that a focus on the actual practice of psychotherapy and the nitty-gritty of what occurs in the therapist's room is of central importance. How do we teach this?

A student at art college has the opportunity of seeing the work of the great artists in front of them, although not the actual process of its creation. But the work of Freud and other pioneers is not there to be seen. We don't really know very well what it was like to be with them in therapy. The best the teacher can do (and this is perhaps most easily done in personal supervision) is to share as openly as possible his or her experiences in therapy without covering up (as is so often done when we write papers) the failings, uncertainties, and the spontaneous ways of behaving which may not appear to be based on sound methodical ideas. For this to happen the structure and culture of the group will have to be directed towards the elimination of superior and inferior status, and that the content of students' discussion groups and seminars could be more focused than they often are on the actual experience of being with patients.

One of the problems of learning psychotherapy is that much of the subject is written in jargon. This is difficult for a beginner to grasp and can be quite intimidating. The student can easily feel the awe which a small child feels in the presence of adults who command fluent speech and use words which to them are obscure. Psychotherapy is, I believe, best communicated in any circumstances by the use of ordinary language insofar as this is possible, and that this eases the path of the student. No other medium of expression has the richness or the resonance to convey the nuances of human intercourse. Of course, simply in order to be able to follow a discussion involving jargon it is desirable at some point that the student should become familiar with the language used (e.g., 'good object,' 'bad object,' and so forth) but this should not be the accepted path to understanding therapy. Unfortunately, as a result of Registration, trainings have been required to show evidence of concentrated focus on one particular theoretical orientation (e.g., 'analytical') resulting in a departure from ordinary language. By contrast, I believe that learning about psychotherapy should involve wide-ranging discussion of cultural issues—of family, society, morality, and so forth—which, if omitted, would lead us too far from the actual world in which we live.

References

1. Evans, Michael (1991), 'Teaching and Learning Psychotherapy,' paper read to Cambridge Society for Psychotherapy.
2. Dewey, John (1956), *The Child and the Curriculum: The School amid Society* University of Chicago Press, p. 9.

Index

Absent father, 3
Action
    feminine, 50–51
    infantile, 49–50
    nature of, 56–57
Adolescent identity crisis, 71
Affects, activity, 49–50
Alienated family, 72
Analytical rationality, 233–234
Anderson, E.W., 95
Assessment, 253–254

Balint, Alice, 185–186
Being and Nothingness (Sartre), 224
Bettleheim, Bruno, 197–198
Binswanger, Ludwig, 217
Blackburn, Thomas, 78–79
Body-mind dichotomy, 183
Bott, Elizabeth, 70, 166
British Independent School, 2, 8
Buber, Martin, 26, 180
Butler, Samuel, 212

Cambridge Psychotherapy Training Group, 238–239
    discussion style, 240–242
    graduation from, 243–246
    selection of new students, 243
    students' work, 242
    theoretical orientation, 239–240
    therapists, 242–243
Cameron, J.L., 130
Castration, 32–33, 157
    childbirth experienced as, 130

Change, 1–2
Child. *See also* Infant
Child, active and passive development of, 53–55
Childbirth. *See also* Puerperal breakdown
    attitude changes of mother during, 91–92
    breakdown after, 4–5
    experienced as castration, 130, 157, 160
    defensive system breakdown at, 142–147
    dread of envy of
        as feminine achievement, 157–158
        as masculine achievement, 158–160
    family study of, 105–123
    Reik's interpretation of, 195–196
    ritual of in primitive societies, 190, 198–199
    Van Gennep's interpretation of, 194–195
Child rearing, 8
    state interference in, 5
Christ-child, 98–99
Circumcision, female, 197–198
Clinical Psychiatry (Mayer-Gross et al), 93
Close-knit families, 71
Clown symbolism, 42
Coates, Stephen, 71
Cohen, A., 193

The Condition of Man (Mumford), 63–64
Conforming family, 120–121
Conversation, 249–250
Cooper, David, 232–234
Countertransference, 250
Couvade, 195–198
Crawley, E., 196
Creative urge, 22–25
Cynicism, 3

Decompensation, 147
Defenses, 7, 225
Denial, 142
Deutsch, Helene, 4, 93, 168
    conception of maternal love, 177–178
Didacticism, 248
Differentiation, lack of, 185
The Divided Self (Laing), 218–219
Dogma, 2
Douglas, G., 93, 135
    on taboo, 207–208
Dreams, 219–220
Dream screen, 37

Educational philosophy, 249
Ego, 230
    boundaries, 27
    feeling, 130–131
    psychology, 216–217
Elite power group, 51
Envy
    dread of, 151–162
    husband's, of childbirth, 196–198
Erewhon (Butler), 212
Erikson, Erik, 8, 130, 211, 217
    on identity, 17, 59, 71, 89
Esterson, A., 231–232
Evans, Michael, 249
Evil father figure, 160
Exhibitionism, 41–42, 152
Existential analysis, 5, 217–218
    and psychoanalysis, 234–235
    on unconscious, 224

Facilitator mother, 123
Fairbairn, W.R.D., 57, 182, 221, 226
False self, 20, 222–223, 225–227
    of schizoid person vs. hysteric, 228
Family, 3
    power dynamics in, 83–85
    relationships in, 63–80
    role of and identity formation, 11–27
    and schizophrenic, 231–232
    state interference in childrearing, 5
    use of sick role in maintaining power balance, 87–88
Family therapy, 6–7
Federn, P., 130, 230
Female
    action of, 50–51
    circumcision of, 197–198
    envy of her creativity, 196–197
    passivity myth, 50–51, 55
    penis envy, 157
    status in society, 76–77
Fenichel, O., 42
Ferenczi, S., 7
Freeman, T., 130
Freud, Anna, 227
Freud, Sigmund, 1–2, 9, 80, 221, 232
    on advantages of illness, 88
    conception of psychoanalysis, 248
    on defenses, 225
    on feminine action, 50
    on impact of family on the child, 65–66
    on infantile action, 49
    on infantile narcissism, 183
    The Interpretation of Dreams, 215
    on object-relationship types, 182
    patriarchal attitude of, 4
    on penis envy in females, 157
    primary and secondary process, 235
    on symptom having meaning, 211
    theory of human growth, 226
    Totem and Taboo, 203–206
    on unconscious, 223
    view of childbirth, 5
Frigidity, 94–96, 142, 166

Giddens, Anthony, 1
God complex, 38–40
Goffman, E., 210
Good father figure, 160
Grandmother role, 151–152
Guilt, 16, 130

Haley, J., 68
Hamilton, J.A., 93

Hartmann, Heinz, 216–217
Haven in a Heartless World (Lasch), 5
Helping professions, 6
Hermann, I., 50–51
Hiroshima, 210
Hoffman, L., 6–7
Home, H.J., 216
Horney, Karen, 157
Horowitz, I.L., 4
Hospital function, 135–136
The House of Elrig (Maxwell), 219–220
Human nature, 2
Husband-wife relationship
    conflict in, 27
    husband's envy of childbirth, 196–198
    during puerperal breakdown, 165–175
Hysteria, 99–100, 228–229

Id, 56–57, 230
Identity, 8
    active and passive, 58–59
    adolescent crisis of, 71, 89
    family role in forming, 11–27
    loss of with schizophrenia, 130, 184
    passivity and failure in forming, 29–60
    sexual, development of, 55–56
I-It relationships, 180
Illness
    primary and secondary gain of, 88
    and taboo, 209–212
    use in maintaining family respectability and meaning, 87–88
Inactivity, 57
Inadequate father, 72–73
Incest, 56
Individual therapy, 6
Individual uniqueness, 2–3
Infant
    action of, 49–50
    idealization of, 131
    narcissism of, 183
    need for self-expression, 76
    passivity of, 52–53
    symbolic meaning of, 160–161
Insanity, fear of, 21–22
The Interpretation of Dreams (Freud), 215

Introjection, 53
Isolation in modern society, 70–71
I-Thou relationships, 180

Jackson, D., 67–68, 86
James, William, 253
Jargon, 255
Jones, Ernest, 158, 206, 215

Kernberg, Otto, 9
Klein, Melanie, 4, 50, 157, 228, 230
    on envy of female creativity, 196–197
    on schizoid person, 220–222

Laing, R.D., 59, 211–212, 223
    The Divided Self, 218–219
    Sanity, Madness, and the Family, 231–232
    on schizoid person, 221–222
    The Self and Others, 234
Langer, M., 157
Lasch, Christopher, 5
Leadership roles, 73–74
Les Rites de Passage (Van Gennep), 194–195
Lewin, Kurt, 234
Lichtenstein, H., 59
Listener, 71
Lomas, P., 55
Loose-knit families, 70–71, 77, 166
Love impulse, 182–183
Lynd, Helen, 130

MacMurray, J., 57
Main, T.F., 85
Male
    status in society, 76–77
    superiority myth, 52
Marx, Karl, 64
Masochism
    of mother, 179–181
    and narcissism, 178–179
    and surrender of child, 161–162
Maternal as concept, 166
Maternal love, 177–178
    difficulty of conceptualizing, 186
    economy of mother-child relationship, 179–181
    mother's perception of her child, 184–186

nature of love impulse, 182–183
relationship between narcissism and masochism, 178–179
Maxwell, Gavin, 219–220
Mayer-Gross, W., 93
McGhie, A., 130
Mental illness, 210
Middle class, 77
Milner, Marion, 23, 185
Modern obstetric practice, 189–200
Moral masochism, 145, 161–162
stages of, 146–147
Mother
facilitator vs. regulator, 123
overpossessive, 72–73
primary preoccupation of, 103, 141, 180, 184–185
professional, 168–169
psychology of, 198–199
of schizophrenic, 98–100
Mother-child relationship, 4
economy of, 179–181
mother's perception of her child, 184–186
narcissism and masochism in, 178–179
"Motherhood and Sexuality" (Deutsch), 168
Mumford, Lewis, 63–64
The Myth of Mental Illness (Szasz), 88

Narcissism
fantasy of, 167–168
of infant, 183
and masochism, 178–179
of object-relationships, 182
Need to be well, 85–87
Nineteen Sixties, 3
Nonpuerperal schizophrenias, 95
Nursing mother, 171

Object-relationships, 182
Object-relations school, 2
Obstetric practice. *See* Modern obstetric practice
Oedipus complex, 25, 32, 56, 66, 196
Overpossessive mother, 72–73

Parasitism, 58
Parental authority, 74–75
Parent-child relationship, 54–55

Parent figure, 26
Parsons, Talcott, 200
Parthenogenetic fantasy, 168–169
Passivity
active and passive development, 53–55
and failure to form identity, 29–49
feminine action, 50–51
of infant, 52–53
infantile action, 49–50
nature of, 57–58
possible reasons for mistaken attributions of, 51–52
Patient, 248
Penis envy, 157, 160
Personal relationships, 232–234
Person perception psychology, 234
Phallus
myth of, 52, 55
symbolism of, 42, 160
Plato, 69
Postmodernism, 1
Power relations, 5
Primary maternal preoccupation, 103, 141, 180, 184–185
Primary process, 235
Primitive societies
and childbirth, 190, 193, 198–199
and taboo, 209
Professional mother, 168–169
Protestant Ethic, 80
Pseudo-mutuality, 19–20, 24, 27
Psychic energy, 229–231
Psychoanalysis
aims of in puerperal breakdown, 137–138
Divided Self of Laing, 218–220
existential, 217–218, 234–235
Freudian, 215–217
hysteria, 228–229
Melanie Klein, 220–222
personal relationships, 232–234
psychic economy, 229–231
retrospective study of family relationships in, 66
schizophrenia and the family, 231–232
true self and false self, 225–227
the unconscious, 223–225
Winnicott, 222–223
Psychoanalyst, 6

Psychodynamic model, 7
Psychosis, 85
Psychotherapy teaching, 247–255
Psychotherapy training, 237
    Cambridge training group, 238–239
    discussion style, 240–242
    graduation from, 243–246
    selection of new students, 243
    students' work, 242
    theoretical orientation, 239–240
    therapists, 242–243
Puerperal breakdown, 4–5, 126–135
    and attitude changes of mother during childbirth, 91–92
    categories of illness, 125–126
    and defensive organization, 141–148
    dread of envy as factor in, 151–162
    hospital function in, 135–136
    husband-wife relationship during, 165–175
    personality defects predisposing women to, 92–104
    psychotherapeutic aims in, 137–138
    therapist function in, 136–137

Queen-Baby, 16

Raphael-Leff, Joan, 123
Reality, 18
Receptivity, 58
Regression to true self, 37, 89
Regulator mother, 123
Reik, Theodore, 195–196
Rites of passage, 194–196, 199–200
Rycroft, C., 37, 57, 230

Sadomasochism, 85, 169
Sanity, 21
Sanity, Madness, and the Family (Laing and Esterson), 231
Sartre, Jean-Paul, 224, 234
Schachtel, E., 49–50, 183, 230
Schizoid
    person, 220–222
    states, 228
Schizophrenic
    and family, 231–232
    loss of identity of, 130, 184
    mother of, 98–100
    primitive wishes of, 131
    pseudo-mutuality in family of, 19–20, 67, 70, 72
Schizophrenogenic family, 14, 122
Scopophilia, 42–44
Searles, Harold F., 18, 56, 85
Secondary process, 235
The Self and Others (Laing), 234
Self-idealization, 75–76
Sense of identity, 8
    effect of family organization on, 17–20
    lack of in schizophrenic families, 184
    recognition of person as unique vs. recognition of person in role, 26–27
Sexual identity, development of, 55–56
Shame, 130
Shaw, George Bernard, 22
Sick family, 27, 70
Sick role, 85
    as temporary therapeutic measure, 88–89
    use in preservation of meaning and respectability, 87–88
Socarides, C.W., 146–147
Social change, 2
Social hierarchy, 74
Sociology, 4
Splitting, 20–22, 182–183
Spontaneous behavior, 36
Stasis, 6–7
Strawson, Galen, 2
Symbiotic parasitism, 14
Symbolic thinking, 235
Symbolic Wounds: Puberty Rites and the Envious Male (Bettleheim), 197
Symbolism
    of baby, 160–161
    of childbirth, 160
    of male exhibitionist, 42
    of passive male, 32–33
    of phallus, 42, 160
Systemic approach, 6–7
Szasz, T.S., 88, 179–180, 211–212, 231

Taboo
    Douglas on, 207–208
    Freud on, 203–206
    on illness, 209–212
    Van Gennep on, 206–207

Teachers, 250
Teaching. *See* Psychotherapy teaching
Technique, 6–7
Therapist, 4, 136–137
Tillich, Paul, 182
Tolstoy, Count Leo, 9
Totem and Taboo (Freud), 203–206
Training. *See* Psychotherapy training
Transference, 6, 131, 224, 234
Transvestism, 42
True self, 20, 37, 161, 222–223, 225–227

Unconscious, 223–225

Van Gennep, Arnold
   interpretation of childbirth, 194–195
   on taboo, 206–207
Victorians, 19

Winnicott, D.W., 4, 20, 93, 211, 228, 230, 248
   on ego boundaries, 27
   on fantasy in narcissistic states, 167
   maternal as concept, 166
   mother's disillusionment in baby, 130
   on primary maternal preoccupation, 103, 141, 180
   on regression to the real self, 37, 89
   on true and false self, 59, 161, 222–223
Witches, 158, 197–198
Wynne, L.C., 19, 184

Zilboorg, G., 93–96, 160, 171